The Appraiser's H

a guide for doctors

Nick Lyons
BSc (Med Sci), MB ChB, MSc (Med Ed), DRCOG, FRCGP

Susanne Caesar
MA (Cantab), MB ChB (Hons), DRCOG, DCH, MRCGP

and

Abayomi McEwen
MBBS (London), MSc (London)

With illustrations by
Sarah Akigbogun

Foreword by
Maurice Conlon

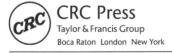

CRC Press
Taylor & Francis Group
Boca Raton London New York

CRC Press is an imprint of the
Taylor & Francis Group, an **informa** business

Radcliffe Publishing Ltd
18 Marcham Road
Abingdon
Oxon OX14 1AA
United Kingdom

www.radcliffe-oxford.com
Electronic catalogue and worldwide online ordering facility.

British Library Cataloguing in Publication Data

A catalogue record for this book is available from the British Library.

ISBN-10: 1 84619 083 5
ISBN-13: 978 1 84619 083 4

Typeset by Anne Joshua & Associates, Oxford

Contents

Foreword

Putting appraisal in the water?

I have read that if the whole population were treated so as to reduce average blood pressure by 2 mmHg, the net benefit in terms of population health gain would be immense. This is partly explained by the inverse care law: those who stand to gain the most from an intervention are the last to whom it is applied.

By making appraisal for doctors a statutory obligation, the NHS has attempted something similar for doctors. Appraisal was lifted out of the domain of enthusiasts and applied to all. This created a challenge: to demonstrate to a profession trained to be scientifically sceptical that appraisal is of value.

One key to this is the proficiency of appraisers. A skilful appraiser can reassure an anxious colleague that appraisal is for their personal benefit, and show a sceptical colleague that appraisal can unlock conundrums which, alone, they have not penetrated.

This book, written by a trio steeped in appraisal, is a valuable resource for appraisers. It will help doctors learning to be appraisers, and experienced appraisers. It will also help those organising appraisal, to remind them of the aims of the process. Teachers of appraisal will be able to use it to supplement and support their curricula.

I believe revalidation, when it arrives, will be the single biggest step towards improvement taken by the profession since the introduction of the medical register. I also believe this depends upon the inclusion of appraisal within the revalidation package. Putting high-quality, developmental appraisal 'in the water' for the medical profession will bring about a whole-profession shift in terms of lifelong professional development. This book will support that aim.

Maurice Conlon FRCGP
Appraisal and Revalidation Lead
NHS Clinical Governance Support Team
www.appraisalsupport.nhs.uk
September 2006

About the authors

Dr Nick Lyons spent a short time in the RAF before training in general practice and settling as a GP in rural Dorset. He gets great fulfilment from his work in medical education, originally as a GP tutor and now as an associate director in Severn and Wessex Deanery. He believes that encouraging and supporting other doctors in their professional development leads to improvements in patient care. He is the appraisal lead for his PCT and works as a member of the editorial team for www.appraisalsupport.nhs.uk. He believes appraisal is at the core of continuing professional development and as vice-chair of the National Association of Primary Care Educators works to raise the profile and quality of education for all those working in primary care.

Dr Susanne Caesar studied in Cambridge and Edinburgh before becoming a GP in Cheshire. She has always enjoyed the variety and wisdom of her patients. Motivated by the desire to make a difference to all GPs, not just the enthusiasts, she has been an appraisal champion since its introduction. Her work as an appraisal training and support provider brings practical experience to this book. The more highly skilled appraisers become, the better they can help motivate individual doctors in their continuing professional development. She gave up a part-time partnership last year in order to have the flexibility to pursue the other branches of her portfolio career, and particularly to have school holidays with her children. In sessional work she has learned the truth that all doctors, no matter where they practise, have something that they can teach others to do better. If, through appraisal, some of this can be captured and shared, she would count it as a major achievement.

Dr Abayomi McEwen was born in Nigeria and inherited her parents' sense of independence and service to society. At the age of 14, her parents sent her to the UK to complete her secondary schooling, and she subsequently trained at the Royal Free Hospital School of Medicine, London University. She gave up her practice in order to devote more time to medical education, specialising in communication and consulting skills. Apart from teaching the teachers, she also works with doctors who have been deemed poorly performing in this area. When appraisal was introduced, the formative and developmental aspect appealed to her natural desire to help others and she gladly accepted the role of Appraisal Lead for Epping Forest PCT. She would like her colleagues to seize appraisal and maximise its potential fully for their benefit and that of their patients. She particularly values the educational input from the National Association of Primary Care Educators in building her knowledge about appraisal. Her family is very important to her and she continues to be truly appreciative of the encouragement her husband, children and extended family give her, even when it means they have to do without her, yet again.

Acknowledgements

The Chinese say 'A journey of a thousand miles starts with one step'. The journey of writing this book has been supported by the encouragement and feedback of many colleagues to whom the authors are genuinely grateful and indebted. Particular mention must go to: John Bibby, Henning Caesar, Maurice Conlon, Julie Draper, Geoff Edwards, Katie Evans, Robin Gleek, Steve Holmes, John Howard, Di Jelley, Keith Judkins, Madeleine Kenny, Peter Leigh, Malcolm Lewis, Anoopam Moar, Bob Royle, Amar Rughani, Stephanie Seiler, Vik Tanna, Jane Whitworth and Dave Young.

The greatest thanks, however, must go to our families, who have tolerated far too many hours of writing and discussions about appraisal. Thank you!

List of abbreviations

BMA	British Medical Association
CME	continuing medical education
CPD	continuing professional development
CRB	Criminal Records Bureau
DEN	doctors' educational needs
DOH	Department of Health
EU	European Union
GMC	General Medical Council
GMS	General Medical Services
GP	general practitioner
GPwSI	general practitioner with a special interest
HPE	higher professional education
IT	information technology
LMC	local medical committee
NAPCE	National Association of Primary Care Educators
NCAS	National Clinical Assessment Service
NCGST	National Clinical Governance Support Team
NHS	National Health Service
NPSA	National Patient Safety Agency
OOH	out of hours
PCT	primary care trust
PDP	personal development plan
PEC	Professional Executive Committee
PEP	phased evaluation project
PGEA	Postgraduate Education Allowance
PPDP	practice professional development plan
PUN	patients' unmet needs
QuOF	Quality and Outcome Framework
RCGP	Royal College of General Practitioners
RITA	Record of In-training Assessment
SCHIN	Sowerby Centre for Health Informatics at Newcastle
SEA	significant event analysis
UK	United Kingdom

For our families

Chapter 1

The purpose of appraisal

This chapter seeks to ensure that the appraiser has a clear understanding of what appraisal is all about.

An understanding of the purpose of appraisal is crucially important to the success of appraisal. Unless the appraiser and the appraisee share the same understanding, then the appraisal discussion is destined to fail.

> To forget one's purpose is the commonest form of stupidity.
> **Friedrich Nietzsche**

The definition of medical appraisal

Appraisal is a confidential developmental process that underpins the doctor's continuing professional development. It seeks to encourage, support and challenge the doctor in delivering the best care to patients through development of the doctor's professional skills, knowledge and attitudes.

Introduction

The introduction of appraisal for doctors has taken place at a time when the position of doctors and other professionals within society is undergoing much change.

The public rightly expects greater accountability, proof of competency and demonstration of high-quality performance than professionals have been accustomed to providing. Precipitated by high-profile cases, perhaps most notably the Shipman murders, the 1990s saw the introduction of clinical governance, the birth of appraisal and the emergence of revalidation.

All these influenced the activity and the continuing professional development of doctors. Some would argue that these changes are for the better, ensuring that doctors are aware of their personal strengths and weaknesses and encouraging them to plan their professional development accordingly. Others feel these changes threaten the very essence of professionalism and that the changes 'dumb down' doctors' development. Doctors spend too much time on meaningless paperwork when they should be using their skills to see patients.

This book aims to support appraisers in developing their skills in order to ensure that the doctor whom they appraise, the appraisee, gains the maximum possible benefit from the time spent in, and preparing for, the appraisal. The appraiser will find appraisees who enthusiastically embrace appraisal and those who doubt its use and place in their professional development. Different approaches may be needed to support and understand different individuals. Certainly all involved in appraisal, both appraisers and appraisees, do need to understand the purpose of appraisal. Research has suggested[1] that poor understanding of this purpose can be a real barrier to the success of appraisal systems. This chapter aims to explore the purpose of appraisal and to consider what an appraisal system is . . . and what it is not.

What is meant by appraisal in society?

Appraisal as a recognised and distinct process, in which the progress and development of the individual is reviewed by an appraiser with that individual, can be traced back over 50 years.[2] Of course, reviewing the progress of an individual in their workplace has been taking place for centuries and is described as long ago as in third-century China.[3]

A review of an individual's ability has always been integral to promotion and success. In organisations as diverse as the Armed Forces, service industries and the mining industry, individuals have been recognised as having ability or potential and have thus been appointed to higher rank, managerial or supervisory positions. It might, however, be argued that some of these promotions have been on the grounds of nepotism rather than individuals' ability or true potential.

What extra dimension does appraisal bring to the process? Appraisal, when done well, aims to look at an individual's abilities and achievements, and seeks to establish an understanding of how the appraisee is motivated to work. Appraisal does not simply leave the review at that stage but looks to understand what qualities and circumstances led to success and how those qualities can be further enhanced and used.

Appraisal seeks to uncover what areas are less easy for, or less well done by, the appraisee and aims to produce a personal plan to help to make changes (either by changing the working experiences of the individual or by equipping them with new skills, new confidence or new attitudes). Appraisal is a dynamic process that looks to help the individuals in their development. It is a catalyst to their personal development.[4]

Appraisal is an ongoing process that encourages individuals to be aware of their strengths and weaknesses, and to identify their developmental needs. The appraisal discussion is just one part of the appraisal process. A well-designed, and well-understood, appraisal process will encourage the individual appraisee to be more thoughtful about their development throughout the year (rather than simply for a few minutes before, during and after the appraisal discussion).

Why then is 'being appraised' not always perceived as the positive opportunity it should be? By the 1980s, appraisal had been adopted by the majority of companies in the United Kingdom but was used in various ways. In some companies it was simply a review of past performance and a mechanism for deciding promotion. In other organisations it was variously used to assess training and developmental needs, set performance objectives and to 'negotiate' future pay increases.[5]

Companies tried to combine a *developmental* review of an individual's strengths and weaknesses with a *performance* assessment, rather than carrying out the appraisal as a separate process,[6] distinct from performance reviews. Some companies tried to link a formative, developmental appraisal discussion with salary reviews and promotion.

It was perhaps not surprising that these attempts encouraged a less than wholehearted revelation of individuals' self-perception of their weaknesses. It was common to find the appraisal was used more as an opportunity to tell people what their manager thought they should be doing[7] rather than looking at individuals' developmental needs and the skills they were capable of offering to the organisation.

Key to the success or failure of appraisal seems to be that the purpose of appraisal needs to be understood by all those involved in it. Appraisal does not work well when different purposes are combined, and works even less well when appraisers are badly trained. There is some evidence that a bad appraisal, as well as leading to dissatisfaction, can actually lead to a decrease in performance and productivity.[8]

There is clearly a tension when considering the purpose of appraisal. If the organisations – the employers – are paying for and supporting the appraisal process, they are entitled to see some return on this investment. If appraisal is all about the individual, rather than the performance of the organisation, can this investment be justified? The answer is probably yes. Senge[9] suggested that the 'learning organisation', where individuals are motivated and encouraged in their personal development, leads to a more efficient and better-performing company. In fulfilling the needs of individuals in the workforce the organisation benefits. This is not simply academic doctrine. There is clear evidence that successful, profitable and growing firms spend more time and money on their employees' personal development[10] than companies with lower levels of achievement.

Inevitably, there will be times when the aims and aspirations of the individual and the company do not coincide. This is not a bar to a successful appraisal; rather the knowledge of this potential conflict allows it to be addressed and is less likely to lead to dissatisfaction and frustration in the longer term.[6]

Appraisal for all?

Appraisal, when done well, leads to a more highly motivated and satisfied workforce.[2] There is a certain irony therefore that individuals in the higher echelons of companies have been slower to adopt appraisal for themselves than they have been to introduce it for their workforce. Furthermore, the lessons learnt in the manufacturing and service industries have only been applied to the public sector in the UK in the past 10 years or so.[2]

The role of the professional, perhaps particularly in the UK, has always been regarded as a 'special case' (not least by the professionals themselves). The professions have been slow to understand and adapt to their changing position in society.

While society still demonstrates great trust in, and respect for, the professions, it now demands that the individual is worthy of that trust and respect. Competence is no longer assumed, rather there is an expectation that it should be demonstrated.

It is against this context that the appraisal of professionals has emerged in the past five years or so, described by Fletcher[2] as a challenging 'new frontier' for appraisal.

The introduction of appraisals for this group of society has not always been easy. Professionals often work in isolation. The complexity of their work means that review of their practice is, in turn, complex and multifactorial.

Individuals may feel that their professional judgement and independence is threatened by the appraisal. Indeed, the driving agenda for the appraisal of professionals working in the public sector has arguably (and reasonably) been to improve the quality of public services. This inevitably means that some individuals will identify the need to engage in significant developments to bring their professional practice to acceptable standards. These changes may often be challenging and difficult to achieve. However, the need for an individual to ensure their continual professional growth is one that true professionalism cannot ignore.

There is some evidence that appraisal for those working in education and other professions has been closer to organisational performance management than a focus on the individual's needs.[11] The professional's suspicion about the introduction of appraisal is therefore not entirely without foundation, yet this relatively privileged and satisfied group of individuals cannot ignore the changes that are expected by the rest of society.[12]

The potential for appraisal as a developmental tool for the individual, a process leading to improvement in performance of both individuals and organisations, seems clear. The application of the process to professionals is relatively recent and has been more challenging. The adoption of appraisal by the medical profession has huge potential. It also presents huge challenges.

Appraisal for doctors

Appraisal for a very few doctors working in the NHS has been taking place successfully for some years.[13] The introduction of a comprehensive appraisal process for all doctors is relatively recent and is without precedent internationally.

At first glance, if one accepts that the advantages perceived in appraisal in industry can be applied to professionals working in medicine, this seems rather odd. After all, the quality of a doctor's work is vitally important to the patient whose life may, literally, be in that doctor's hands. It also important to the health service that resources the investigations and treatment the doctor provides. One should also remember that the introduction of appraisal to the management systems of large organisations is challenging,[14] and that the introduction of appraisal for professionals is a yet more demanding task.

It is understandable therefore that a national appraisal system for all doctors began to be introduced only as recently as 2001. It is a great credit to those involved in developing the appraisal process that is has been so rapidly integrated into the professional life of every NHS doctor across the UK.

Pilot schemes for more formal appraisal processes were developed in the 1980s and 1990s in secondary,[15] community[16] and primary care.[17] These involved a very small minority of doctors and lagged far behind similar systems in the nursing profession, both in the uptake of appraisal and in the understanding of the benefits and purposes of appraisal.[18]

The pilot appraisal systems for doctors and the more established systems for nurses shared, in common with industry, the problems and uncertainties generated by confusion about the purpose of appraisal.[16,19] There was a perception by some, but by no means all, that appraisal was more about the performance management of individuals than about their personal development.

The majority of doctors in the late 1990s did not have an annual appraisal. Their continuing professional development involved participation in various educational programmes of continuing medical education (CME) administered by the Royal Colleges or, in the case of GPs, attendance at educational events accredited by tutors employed by deaneries and leading to the payment of a Postgraduate Education Allowance (PGEA).

The majority of this educational activity was probably good. Some, indeed, was very good. However, other education was undoubtedly poor.[20] Although the advantages of personal development plans to focus and direct professional development were accepted in medical education circles,[21] there was little, if any, compulsion to participate and produce such a plan. In the late 1990s came acceptance that continuing professional development (CPD) needed management and leadership to become more effective in supporting and developing professionals to give high-quality care to patients.[22]

The widening professional concern about the quality of CPD, and strengthening impetus to manage and improve this activity, coincided with the media and public outcry generated, with great justification, by the infamous Bristol paediatric heart surgery scandal. The murders committed by Dr Harold Shipman in general practice brought the deficiencies in the regulation of doctors further into public discussion.

The medical profession's place in society was changed forever, and the trust of the public to allow doctors to self-regulate and be responsible for the structure and management of their own professional development was over. Sadly, many professionals failed, and some still do fail, to recognise that while these cases may have been aberrant, the goalposts for developing as an individual professional had moved.

Clinical governance came of age while this media hysteria raged, but there was also a growing and more measured concern among many in society that these cases exposed genuine flaws in the ability of the medical profession to self-regulate and to monitor the professional practice of doctors.

The introduction of clinical governance was perhaps more easily adopted than many had predicted, no doubt eased by the involvement of large numbers of doctors in the management structures of the early primary care groups and acute trusts. This led to a more open culture of audit, the wider use of significant event analysis and performance markers, and an acceptance that addressing the poor performance of an individual practitioner was a collective responsibility.

Revalidation of doctors, and reaccreditation of their specialist skills, became accepted as a desirable element of doctors' regulation and the General Medical Council (GMC) began radical changes in its organisation, with increased openness and lay involvement. It also, in 1998, began the long, and very winding, road towards the agreement of a model of revalidation that could be effective and reliable, as well as being acceptable to the demands of the government, the public and the professions.[23]

In retrospect, it is perhaps surprising therefore that the government launched its proposals for appraisal for consultants in 2001 with a firm emphasis on supporting the 'learning and personal development needs for consultants'[24] rather than proposing it as a performance management tool. The temptation must have been there to use appraisal as a tool to manage doctors, force their compliance with organisational changes and direct their development to the needs of the organisation. Instead, the guidance wisely chose to follow the principles of Senge's learning organisation[9] and focus on the needs of the individual.

Despite the clear guidance that this was a formative process aimed at the individual doctor, confusion about the purpose of appraisal among those doctors facing appraisal for the first time was rife. The confusion was mirrored in some areas by those developing and carrying out appraisals, and led to much consternation for some doctors.[25] Others challenged the profession (and many of the experiences of the non-medical world) and suggested that appraisal could effectively be used for the twin purposes of performance management and formative personal development.[26]

Appraisal for general practitioners began to be rolled out a year later, in 2002, with very similar guidance notes to those for consultants, the emphasis being on the development of the individual GP. The emphasis on review of their performance was slightly more overt for GPs than it had been for consultants.[27,28] Initially aimed at GP principals, the process was further extended to include all GPs in 2004.[29]

The early uptake of general practice appraisal, the cynical might argue, was high because in the early stages it was relatively well funded. The vast majority of GPs joined in the process. Research suggests it was found to be useful and surprisingly well received.[30] Confusion about the purpose of appraisal inevitably persisted in a similar way as for consultants.

If appraisal for established doctors was introduced between 2001 and 2004, appraisal for doctors in training had existed (arguably not comprehensively) for many years. The Record of In-training Assessment (RITA)[31] had great potential to be a formative developmental tool, but, again, attempts to combine formative development with career-important summative assessment undermined the process for many. It is interesting to note that the appraisal of doctors in training is now slowly becoming a more formative process. The assessment tools evident in Modernising Medical Careers[32] may further strengthen appraisal as a developmental tool for trainees.

It is a real testimony to the enthusiasm of the appraisers and the managers tasked with introduction of the appraisal process for doctors that, in less than three years, the concept of a developmental appraisal could move from being the domain of a few enthusiasts to a widespread process that has been largely accepted by the majority of doctors. Appraisal appears to be slowly and effectively altering the learning behaviour and attitudes of doctors. While appraisal for professionals has been recognised as a challenging area, the UK medical profession has integrated it within professional practice with remarkable speed and enthusiasm. Those critical of the inertia of the profession should perhaps consider carefully the evidence for their concerns.

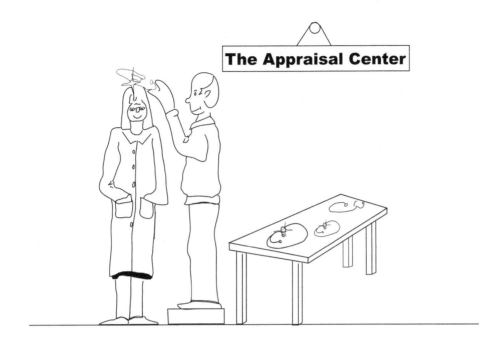

WE AIM TO MAKE YOU A BETTER DOCTOR

What appraisal for doctors is . . . and is not

It is sad that, despite the clear intention that appraisal for doctors should be a developmental process that seeks to encourage and support the doctor, it should be approached with trepidation by many doctors.

Why? There is certainly concern about the purpose of the appraisal and we have seen that this is a valid issue in all appraisal systems, not simply those for doctors. Judgement of a doctor's performance cannot always be effectively combined with honest disclosure and objective discussion by that doctor about their developmental needs.

The most significant worries and concerns individual doctors have, the most important to be discussed in the protected, confidential arena of appraisal, will be hidden if appraisees feel this might affect their career prospects and their income.

Even within a purely developmental appraisal there is, for many, a natural resistance to talking about their needs. Traditional medical training has, for many, been akin to the ritual humiliation meted out by James Robertson Justice in *Doctor in the House*.[33] An honest disclosure of need is often seen as being an admittance of unacceptable weakness, a concept alien to doctors whose professional defences were shaped in traditional medical schools.

Appraisal is not about judging the doctor's performance; it is not about measuring performance against a trust's targets. It is, however, part of a process that encourages the doctor to look at their own professional practice on a regular basis and to consider how that practice can be improved. It is the application of the skills of the reflective practitioner.[34] The appraisal process does not simply require the doctor to reflect on their activities on an annual basis as a preparation for the appraisal interview, rather it encourages 'reflection-in-action' so that the doctor adopts a more thoughtful approach to their practice, and the effects of that practice on others, as a part of their day-to-day professional lives. Creating reflective practitioners will benefit the individual, the organisation and patients.

A judgemental, destructive, performance-based appraisal may be feared and is not a part of the appraisal process as laid out for doctors in the NHS. A developmental appraisal that indulges the appraisee in their reflections without challenge is equally wrong and is likely to prove a waste of time for the appraiser and the appraisee. The good appraiser will ensure that neither extreme occurs.

The appraisal discussion provides an opportunity for challenge and for objective discussion to determine the real developmental needs of the appraisee. It allows an outside and objective view of the personal world of the individual doctor's development and is likely to be successful only if the appraiser enjoys the trust and the respect of that doctor.

The skill of the appraiser lies in determining whether to challenge the complacency of the doctor and encourage them to accept their imperfections and produce a realistic development plan that will address some of those needs. All this needs to be done without adding to the doctor's stress and insecurity.

It does need to be remembered that the appraiser is there to look forwards as well as backwards. There needs to be an agreement on the developmental needs of the doctor. This can certainly involve both challenge and encouragement, but the appraiser also needs to help the doctor to turn needs into developmental objectives, identifying how the doctor can find effective and relevant educational activity.[35] The appraiser needs to gain an understanding of how doctors learn in order to help them in their production of an effective personal development plan.

The appraiser, if effective, and if allowed to do so by the appraisee, enters personal territory. It is important that both parties appreciate that they are there to look at the doctor's development. The appraiser is not the appraisee's doctor, his counsellor or his psychologist. Nor is the appraiser the priest or the teacher. While this may seem so obvious that it does not need recording, it is when appraisals stray into these areas, as they often do, that appraisers need to be sure of their role.

This is perhaps a more real problem when appraisers may, in the rest of their professional lives, routinely use counselling, teaching or psychological skills and thus may not easily recognise when they leave appraisal territory to enter more complicated waters. The caring and conscientious appraiser may also struggle to leave problems that have been identified to be addressed by others later. Most appraisers will admit to sometimes being tempted to becoming involved in the personal support of the doctor beyond the normal arena of appraisal, and perhaps this is inevitable, if not without danger. The central purpose of appraisal, the developmental support of the individual in his professional life, must not be forgotten.

Appraisal is a more complex process than it may first appear. Its structure depends on both the appraiser and the appraisee and also the context within which the appraisal is taking place. It relies on the trust of the appraisee and the skills of the appraiser, and depends on both sharing the same understanding of the purpose of the exercise.

An effective appraisal process does not simply involve a successful appraisal discussion. The preparation for the appraisal and the actions that follow it are also determinants of success and should lead to an ongoing upward spiral of development where, year on year, there is review of a doctor's development and production of short-, medium- and long-term developmental priorities and actions.

The appraisal discussion catalyses[4] that process on an annual basis, giving fresh impetus, challenge and encouragement to the doctor. As the years pass, the appraisee should become better equipped to examine their own strengths and weaknesses and should be increasingly able to consider how to direct their professional development, hence leading to better care for their patients, colleagues and themselves.

References

1   Lewis M, Elwyn G, Wood F. Appraisal of family doctors: an evaluation study. *Br J Gen Pract*. 2003; **53**(491): 454–60.
2   Fletcher C. *Appraisal: routes to improved performance*. 2nd ed. London: Institute of Personnel and Development; 1997.
3   Swan W. *How To Do a Superior Performance Appraisal*. New York: Wiley Books; 1991.
4   Conlon M. Appraisal: the catalyst to personal development. *BMJ*. 2002; **327**: 389–91.
5   Long P. *Performance Appraisal Revisited*. London: Institute of Personnel Management; 1986.
6   Meyer H, Kay E, French J. Split roles in performance appraisal. *Harvard Bus Rev*. 1965; **43**: 123–9.
7   Dulewicz V, Fletcher C. The context and dynamics of performance appraisal. In: Heriot P, editor. *Assessment and Selection in Organisations*. London: John Wiley; 1989.
8   Murphy K, Cleveland JN. *Understanding Performance Appraisal*. London: Sage; 1995.
9   Senge P. *The Fifth Discipline: the art and practice of the learning organisation*. London: Random House; 1990.
10   Harvard B. *Performance Appraisals*. London: Kogan Page; 2001.
11   Bartlett S. The development of teacher appraisal: a recent history. *Br J Educ Stud*. 2000; **48**: 24–8.
12   Exworthy M *et al*. The role of performance indicators in challenging the autonomy of the general practice profession in the UK. *Soc Sci Med*. 2003; **56**: 1493–504.
13   Chambers R *et al*. *The Good Appraisal Toolkit for Primary Care*. Oxford: Radcliffe Medical Press; 2004.
14   Edmonstone J. Appraising the state of performance appraisal. *Health Manpower Manage*. 1996; **6**: 9–13.
15   Giddins G, Turner J. Personnel appraisal. *Br J Health Care Manage*. 1995; **1**(2): 82–6.
16   Horn N, Pullan C. Appraisal system for community child health doctors. *Public Health*. 1996; **110**: 103–5.
17   Haman H, Irvine S, Jelley D. *The Peer Appraisal Handbook for General Practitioners*. Oxford: Radcliffe Medical Press; 2001.
18   Edis M. *Performance Management and Appraisal in Health Services*. London: Kogan Page; 1995.
19   Hale C. Providing support for nurses in general practice through clinical supervision: a key element of the clinical governance framework. *J Clin Gov*. 1999; **7**: 162–4.
20   Richards T. Continuing medical education. *BMJ*. 1998; **316**(7127): 246.

21 Challis M. AMEE Medical Education Guide 19: Personal Learning Plans. *Med Teach.* 2000; **22**(3): 225–36.

22 Grant J, Chambers E, Jackson G. *The Good CPD Guide: a practical guide to managed CPD.* Sutton: The Joint Centre for Education in Medicine; 1999.

23 Chief Medical Officer. *Good Doctors, Safer Patients.* London: DoH; 2006.

24 Department of Health. *NHS Appraisal: appraisal for consultants working in the NHS.* London: DoH; 1999.

25 Kerr D. Political correctness is behind proposed appraisal system. *BMJ.* 1999; **318**(7189): 1013a.

26 Taylor CM, Wall DW, Taylor CL. Appraisal of doctors: problems with terminology and a philosophical tension. *Med Educ.* 2002; **36**(7): 667–71.

27 Department of Health. *NHS Appraisal: guidance on appraisal for general practitioners working in the NHS.* London: DoH; 2002.

28 Martin D *et al. Appraisal for GPs.* Sheffield: University of Sheffield, School of Health and Related Research (ScHARR); 2001.

29 Martin D, Harrison P, Joesbury H. *Extending Appraisal to All GPs.* Sheffield: University of Sheffield, School of Health and Related Research (ScHARR); 2003.

30 Denney M. Annual appraisal: where have we got to? *Educ Primary Care.* 2005; **16**: 697–703.

31 Riley W. Appraising appraisal. *BMJ.* 1998; **317**(7170): 2.

32 Chief Medical Officer. *Unfinished Business: proposals for reform of the Senior House Officer Grade.* London: DoH; 2003.

33 Thomas R. *Doctor in the House.* Carlton Entertainment; 1954.

34 Schon D. *The Reflective Practitioner: how professionals think in action.* 2nd ed. Aldershot: Arena; 1991.

35 Brookfield S. *Understanding and Facilitating Adult Learning.* Buckingham: Open University Press; 1986.

Chapter 2

Appraisal and professional development

> This chapter looks at the basics of appraisal and what the appraiser is trying to achieve. It considers the appraisal process in the context of the wider professional development of doctors.

Life is about learning; when you stop learning, you die.

Tom Clancy

Doctors and learning

The doctor has an incredibly important and complex role in society. Doctors are expected to behave and act in a responsible way and to be trustworthy and reliable.

The doctor has a detailed knowledge of complex issues based on a sound scientific understanding and application of basic clinical sciences. This knowledge, acquired in secondary school and medical school, of how the human body works and what happens to make it go wrong, is refined and developed over years to allow the doctor to diagnose, treat and support patients. As doctors develop in their training they learn the art of professional judgement, tailoring treatment to the physical, psychological, emotional and spiritual needs of an individual patient.

Doctors develop sophisticated interpersonal skills to enable them to gather information from patients and to explain treatments to those same patients, who may not share any of the doctor's scientific training and language.

Complex practical skills are gained by doctors, enabling them to carry out intricate surgical procedures and use sophisticated machinery and equipment in their day-to-day practice. They are often seen as leaders and managers, with responsibility for large departments and budgets as well as the planning and development of medical services to reflect the needs of the local population.

The professional development of doctors needs to support them in their careers and respond to their needs. These needs will not be the same for any two doctors, as individuals' knowledge, skills and attitudes will vary, as will their professional responsibilities, career aims and career aspirations.

Doctors, then, must surely be sophisticated learners who are able to identify and successfully respond to their learning needs. To achieve all that they achieve, this must be so. However, it seems to be in spite of, rather than because of, much of their medical education.[1]

Some doctors fail to see the relevance of much of their education in medical school. They look back on their training as junior doctors in hospital with a certain horror. They sometimes also find it difficult to prioritise and identify their learning needs in their continuing professional development as established doctors.

They may not be able to use time spent learning effectively and many tend to concentrate on the areas of continuing medical education that they find interesting (which are often already areas of strength) rather than the areas where they need to develop their knowledge, skills and attitudes to enable them to care better for their patients.

Doctors are usually (but arguably not always) reasonably intelligent individuals and it may be that they have evolved methods of learning that intuitively work for them. It is certainly true that the doctor's workplace is a rich learning environment. There are always opportunities to learn from patients and colleagues. However, with the speed of development of medical knowledge increasing all the time, the changing role of doctors within the National Health Service and the need to respond to the needs and expectations of patients, it seems unlikely that learning that takes place 'in action' is going to be sufficient. There needs to be a system for doctors to consider what gaps there may be in their knowledge, skills and attitudes, and reliable and efficient ways to address the needs identified.

Adults and learning

How do adults learn? The appraiser does not need a degree in adult learning theory to appraise effectively, but an understanding of some of the basic principles may be useful.

There are various schools of thought about the theories surrounding learning. If these are blended together, it is possible to construct a pragmatic view that is useful to the appraiser.

One school of educational thought, behaviourism, proposes that we are all driven by objectives and that we learn best in multiple small and clearly defined steps. The humanist focuses more attention on the individual learner and his feelings, and argues that we learn most effectively when the learning is relevant to our needs.

Adult learning theory suggests that we learn better when we are motivated and see benefit in what we are learning. As we mature from dependent child learners to experienced adult learners, learning is increasingly seen in the context of our past experiences, and these experiences are essential to us in translating our learning into practice.

Some may find it helpful to think of this in terms of a learning cycle where we continually experience new ideas and then think about them and apply them to practice, checking to see whether our 'hypotheses' are correct. This process, whereby knowledge is built on experience, is variously attributed but often termed Kolb's Learning Cycle (Figure 2.1).[2]

Some learning activity is effective, whereas other activity probably is not. It is important that doctors, as busy professionals with waiting lists and performance targets, spend time on learning that 'works' and less time on activity that does little for their development.

Rogers[3] and Freiburg suggested 10 principles of learning that can help to ensure that learning is effective, and some of these are useful for the appraiser to consider (Box 2.1).

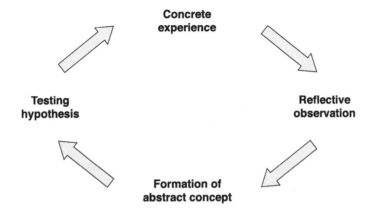

Figure 2.1 Kolb's Learning Cycle.

Box 2.1 Rogers and Freiburg's principles of learning

1 Human beings have a natural potential to learn
2 Learning is most effective when the learner sees it as relevant to their lives
3 Learning involving change, particularly to oneself, tends to be resisted
4 Learning that does involve change and threat is more easily assimilated when other threats are at a minimum
5 When threat to oneself is low, learning proceeds most effectively
6 Significant learning is often done through doing
7 Learning works best when the learner is actively involved in the learning process
8 Self-initiated learning is the most effective
9 Independence and creativity works best when external evaluation is not intrusive
10 The most important learning is learning about learning

It makes sense for appraisers to help doctors understand how they learn and how to spend their time learning to the greatest effect. If they participate in workshops, attend lectures or read journals that are relevant to their working lives and their needs, if they are actively involved in that learning and if they recognise that within themselves there may be a tendency to resist change, even change that is needed, Carl Rogers would suggest that they are more likely to gain from the experience than if they attend random educational events in which they participate little.

The interested reader can find many books that explore adult education theory in detail,[4,5] but there are a few other ideas that appraisers may find useful to keep at the back of their minds when considering how appraisal relates to change and motivation of the individual.

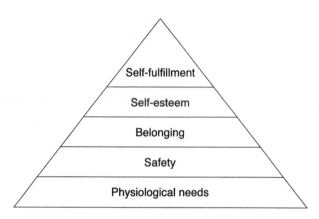

Figure 2.2 Maslow's Pyramid.

The environment of learning

Maslow was an American psychologist who described a hierarchy of needs.[6] At the most simplistic, Maslow would say that if we are cold, hungry and tired we are less likely to learn effectively than if we are in comfortable surroundings, uninterrupted and with time available to think about our learning. The other lesson for the appraiser is that there is little point talking to doctors about self-fulfilment (or self-actualisation, as Maslow termed it) if they feel bullied and exposed in the workplace or they or their family are facing illness or other problems. The foundations have to be right if learners are going to be able to move on in their professional development (Figure 2.2).

Needs and learning

It is not difficult to agree with Rogers that learning is likely to be most effective when it is relevant to the needs of the learner. We have already looked at Kolb's Learning Cycle, where learning is experienced and then considered, applied and tested in the real world.[2]

Somewhat confusingly, there are several other 'learning cycles' and the authorship of one of the most useful is unclear.[7] This learning cycle is summarised in Figure 2.3.

The doctor will have some areas that he does not know he doesn't know ('unconscious incompetence'). Once these have been identified as developmental needs, they are known and the doctor is aware of them ('conscious incompetence'). The doctor then addresses the needs and may have to think at first about the application of the new knowledge or skills ('conscious competence') but, as with the learner driver once they have learned how to operate the clutch, these new abilities soon become second nature ('unconscious competence').

Interestingly, and poorly researched or described in the literature, those skills may decay or new standards for practice emerge and thus the doctor may slip from 'unconscious competence' to 'unconscious *in*competence' at varying rates. This is

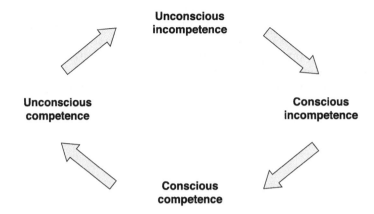

Figure 2.3 The learning cycle.

clearly a part of this learning cycle. It is the recognition of this stage, worrying for patient care, that is one of the fundamental building blocks of the appraisal process.

Another way of looking at this is to consider Johari's Window,[8] which considers learning needs from a different perspective (Figure 2.4). If both the appraiser and the appraisee know of a developmental need, then useful discussion about that need can take place in the 'open agenda' of the appraisal.

It is possible that the appraisee may know of a need that they choose not to discuss in the appraisal. While such 'hidden agendas' may not always be of great importance, if they are of significant relevance to professional development this could be of some concern and might call into question how genuinely the appraisee is participating in the appraisal process.

If appraisers identify from the material they are given prior to appraisal, or from issues that arise during the appraisal discussion, that there is a need that is not seen by the doctor, this 'blind spot' in the view of the doctor being appraised needs to be handled carefully. With skill it may be brought into the arena of the 'open agenda' or, using the learning cycle model, from unconscious to conscious incompetence. This does assume that the appraiser is capable of assessing the needs of the doctor better than they are themselves. This may be a dangerous assumption.

	Known to self (appraisee knows)	Unknown to self (appraisee does not know)
Known to others (appraiser knows)	Open agenda	Blind spot
Unknown to others (appraiser does not know)	Hidden agenda	No agenda

Figure 2.4 Johari's Window for appraisal.

The bottom right area of Johari's Window is uncharted territory (unknown to appraiser and appraisee) which may, or may not, be significant. The skilled appraiser aims to bring as many of the issues relevant to the doctor's development as possible into the 'open agenda', but must recognise that the other areas may exist. These sometimes appear when least expected.

Over time it should be hoped that the amount of information in the 'unknown' box diminishes as the appraisee becomes more adept at identifying his needs and reflecting on his development.

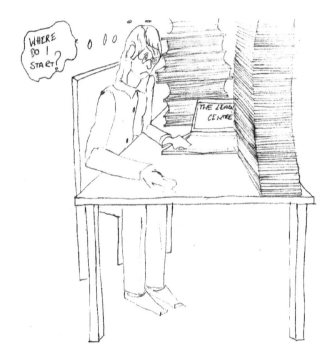

Appraisal and learning

It is important that appraisees and appraisers alike see appraisal as a part of the bigger picture of continuing professional development. It certainly can be the catalyst to personal development[9] and lies at the heart of professional development.

The appraisal discussion is a tool to look at the appraisee's needs and assist in prioritising those needs in the context of professional practice. The preparation for the appraisal and the action that follows on from the appraisal are just as, if not more, important than the appraisal itself and serve to lead the learning doctor around the educational cycles and through the stages of learning described in this chapter.

The appraisal is an active process and involves challenge and rigour, but also support and encouragement to try and bring all doctors to their full potential: the self-actualisation of Maslow's Pyramid.

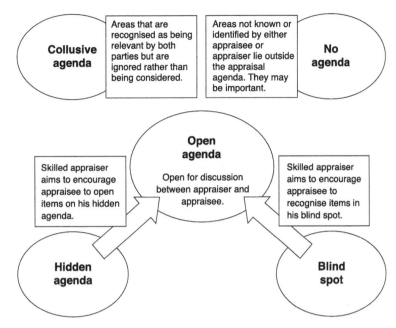

Figure 2.5 The Yosuni Appraisal Windows.

The Yosuni Windows

Using the image of windows, the Yosuni Appraisal Windows are laid out in Figure 2.5. The central area for discussion about the appraisee's development is the 'open agenda'. This lies at the centre of the appraisal process and is where the appraiser considers with the appraisee how they can develop their practice to better look after patients, work with colleagues and look after themselves, all in the context of their own professional development.

There will be areas that doctors may not feel they need, or wish, to discuss with the appraiser. These describe the 'hidden agenda'. The appraisee leads the agenda for appraisal, but the skilled appraiser will try and ensure that all important areas are available for discussion. It is the critical reading of the pre-appraisal documentation and excellent communication skills that will ensure the success or failure of bringing the 'hidden agenda' into the open.

Blind spots are inevitable for all of us and should not be seen as failures in the appraisee. Rather, bringing these areas of potential 'unconscious incompetence' into the open agenda is an important, and inevitable, part of learning (although it may need a skilled facilitative appraiser to do the job well).

The areas that may not as easily enter the appraisal process are the 'collusive agenda' and the 'no agenda'. The collusive agenda, described in Yosuni's window, may remain outside the appraisal, but with a self-aware, honest and skilled appraiser, and an appraisee who trusts the system, this becomes less likely. True collusion represents a real danger to an effective appraisal process as areas of genuine concern may not be addressed.

The 'unknown unknowns' are reduced by bringing the blind, the hidden and the collusive into the open agenda. The 'no agenda' will become smaller. While the appraisal process may minimise this by using tools that work to identify learning and developmental needs that are unknown, it can never eliminate the 'no agenda' completely.

The ideas expressed in this section are fundamental to effective adult learning. Appraisal for doctors is, in turn, fundamental to effective professional development.

> Appraisal is a confidential developmental process that underpins the doctor's continuing professional development. It seeks to encourage, support and challenge the doctor in delivering the best care to patients through development of the doctor's professional skills, knowledge and attitudes

Learning styles: we are all different

Doctors share many common traits but have a great variety of needs. How they address these needs will depend partly on the way they learn, and here too there are differences, both between doctors and also at different times for the same doctor. There are many classifications and attempts to better understand our characters which may help us to gain insights into our strengths and weaknesses[10] and these may be worthy of exploration.[11]

In relation to learning, there are particular descriptions of learning styles, the best known of which are perhaps those developed by Peter Honey and Alan Mumford.[12] They describe learning style preferences that significantly affect the way we learn:

- activist
- reflector
- theorist
- pragmatist.

These styles are expressed in us all, but the degrees of expression vary between individuals and also in ourselves according to the arena in which we are learning. The categories are self-explanatory and, despite work questioning the value of learning styles,[13] they feel intuitively reasonable. The activist will jump into learning before the more measured reflector. The theorist has to understand the topic fully and will clarify details that the pragmatist will see as distracting.

Appraisees can be encouraged to identify their own learning styles and use the insight gained to plan their learning activity.

The key message for the appraiser is that we may all learn differently and that what is right for the appraiser may not be right for the appraisee.

Development plans

The appraisal interview should always be summarised and carefully recorded. In medical appraisal in the UK this is done on Form 4, a simple document that is laid out by the Department of Health.[14,15] This basic format has been adapted and developed in various parts of the UK.[16,17]

Within the documentation lies a personal development template (sometimes termed 'the grid'). It is probably fair to say that this has not always been completed with great thought or in much detail. What is the purpose of this template? What is the evidence that it serves any purpose if the rest of the Form 4 already summarises the appraisal interview?

While the terminology is sometimes confusing, there is significant evidence that summarising and planning one's learning is a useful process and is more likely to lead to activity that is useful for the learner.[18,19] It could be argued that the activity inherent in development planning is the same as that in the whole of the appraisal process. This is indeed so, but the development plan serves to allow the appraisee time to reflect on what has been said. It ensures (if they fill the development plan out themselves) that the appraiser is not stamping their own agenda on the appraisee's learning and allows time to reflect on what has been said in the appraisal discussion.

The appraiser and the appraisee who neglect the importance of the development plan risk losing that part of the process that encourages the doctor to move from passive to active ownership of their learning agenda.

The effectiveness of appraisal

Does appraisal make a difference? There is ample evidence that it is enjoyed and is felt to be worthwhile,[20–22] although very little evidence[23] that it actually makes a difference to the way doctors conduct their learning and professional development.

This lack of concrete evidence may seem surprising, but it reflects the difficulty of research in this area. Indeed, there is little evidence that any continuing professional development makes a difference to patient care.[24,25]

Complex outcomes are notoriously difficult to evaluate and therein lies a challenge to appraisers and educators to conduct research to demonstrate what does, and does not, make for effective educational practice.

The areas covered in appraisal

Appraisal is designed to look at all aspects of a doctor's professional development. The initial work on doctors' appraisal[26,27] showed the need to give this comprehensive overview, and the official guidance and documentation bears this out.[14,15]

The categories of appraisal are derived from the General Medical Council (GMC) document that describes the duties and responsibilities of doctors, *Good Medical Practice*,[28] and for GPs also draws on a more comprehensive publication, *Good Medical Practice for General Practitioners*.[29]

While the terminology varies slightly and the order in which they are laid out is different, the scope of the appraisal is the same for all doctors (perhaps unsurprisingly as both systems are derived from the same document) (Table 2.1).[30,31]

What do these areas mean? They should together provide a comprehensive look at a doctor's practice, enabling the appraisee to reflect on all aspects of his

Table 2.1 Areas covered in appraisal for consultants and GPs

Consultants	General practitioners
Good medical care	Good clinical care
Maintaining good medical practice	Maintaining good medical practice
Working relationships with colleagues	Relationships with patients
Relations with patients	Working with colleagues
Teaching and training	Teaching and training
Probity	Probity
Health	Management activity
Management activity	Research
Research	Health

professional work. Interestingly, and perhaps unfortunately, nowhere does the guidance specifically encourage the doctor to look at their professionalism, that sometimes ill-defined and much misunderstood quality that is so important to the effective and respected doctor. A recent working party suggested[32] that this should be more clearly stated as the theme that runs through the whole appraisal.

> Medicine is a vocation in which a doctor's knowledge, clinical skills and judgement are put in the service of protecting and restoring human well-being. This purpose is realised through a partnership between patient and doctor, one based on mutual respect, individual responsibility, and appropriate accountability.
>
> **Royal College of Physicians**[32] (p.14)

There is some confusion at times among both appraisees and appraisers as to what topics should be considered in each section. Careful reading of the explanatory notes that accompany the appraisal paperwork clarifies much of the confusion, and this is helped further if the appraisee has a clear understanding of appraisal gained through workshops, from colleagues, local support packs or by reading one of the excellent books published to help in preparation for appraisal.[33–35]

It may be helpful, however, to think of 'Good Medical/Clinical Care' as looking at how individuals show that they provide a good standard of care to their patients and how that clinical care can be strengthened. It is the area where variance from ideal care may first be recognised and discussed.

This complements the following section, 'Maintaining Good Medical Practice', where the emphasis is on how the doctor identifies his learning needs and then organises and participates in professional development activity. There are clear overlaps between the sections as needs cannot be defined until there has been some benchmarking and consideration of what is going well, and what may be going less well. If the appraiser encourages the doctor to organise thoughts, paperwork and planning, much angst (and duplication of effort) may be avoided.

The remaining sections are no less important but are more self-explanatory. The appraiser needs to ensure all areas are considered (and how this is best done is the subject of other chapters of this book) but may well not conduct the appraisal discussion in the strict order that topics appear on the paperwork.

The skilled appraiser will be picking up on issues as they arise in the discussion and the challenge is to ensure that important areas are not neglected if they arise in an order inconvenient for the appraiser's train of thought, but crucial to the needs of the appraisee.

The evidence informing appraisal

The appraisal must be based on factual information and the doctor's reflection on the important lessons to be learnt from that information. This is not an easy skill to acquire and is not intuitive for everybody.[36] The appraisee needs to think carefully about the material provided for appraisal and the appraiser needs to develop critical reading skills in looking at this material.

We now start to enter choppy waters. The purpose of the appraisal is to encourage the doctor in their development; it is not about performance assessment. How then should the appraisee use information and how can the appraiser assess the material? The key is to remember that the information is there to support a discussion about the doctor's development. To do that effectively the appraiser needs to encourage the appraisee to consider what lessons can be learnt from audit material, for example.

The material submitted to inform the appraisal discussion has been termed 'evidence' in much of the appraisal and revalidation paperwork. This immediately introduces a legalistic flavour to proceedings which need not be there. It might be better termed 'supporting information' reflecting the relationship of the 'evidence' to the appraisal process.

Examples of documentation and evidence that may inform the appraisal discussion are laid out to help the appraisee and the appraiser ensure that a sufficiently wide view of practice is obtained. It is important to ensure that these are not seen as a checklist of documentation that must be submitted by all doctors in all situations every year. Instead, the portfolio of evidence that supports appraisal should develop into a comprehensive view over time of the doctor's professional activity, which examines all aspects of the care they provide to patients and the wider aspects of their professional role. To avoid duplication of effort and needless 'hoop jumping', this portfolio should also contain any specific evidence required for revalidation.

The appraiser has a role in spotting 'missing evidence' and helping the appraisee to think of ways to plug any holes. This support is perhaps particularly important when appraising sessional doctors in general practice and locum doctors in the hospital setting, where comprehensive data on clinical activity and prescribing may not be present and where true audit is often impossible. The problem of obtaining evidence also applies to many doctors working in managed environments where the data that is available is insufficiently detailed or analysed to be 'fit for purpose' in informing appraisal.

The appraiser assesses the information submitted in appraisal for its fitness to inform the appraisal discussion rather than using the paperwork to attempt to carry out a performance assessment of the doctor. Such performance assessment is important but needs different skills and training and is distinct from appraisal. It is nonetheless vitally important that if an appraiser uncovers evidence of poor performance, or has a concern that the doctor may be in difficulty, that this is dealt with. Indeed, this is a responsibility incumbent on all doctors at all times.

> You must protect patients when you believe that a doctor's or other colleague's health, conduct or performance is a threat to them.
>
> **General Medical Council**[28] (p.9)

While all doctors should understand this responsibility, it does need to be made explicit to the appraisee. This is discussed in more detail in Chapter 5.

Appraisal and revalidation

The critical reading of the supporting information for appraisal reminds the appraiser of the purpose of appraisal. The link between appraisal and revalidation takes the appraiser into stormy and uncharted waters.

Revalidation is a relatively new concept and was born out of the controversies and concerns of society in the 1990s as described in Chapter 1 of this book. It is a fundamentally different process from appraisal and seeks to ensure the doctor's fitness to practice.[37] Revalidation will probably require the doctor to participate in appraisal and the challenge may well be in defining what 'participate' means.

As this book goes to press the debate about the relationship between appraisal and revalidation continues,[38] but some guiding principles can be stated with reasonable confidence.

There is no reason why the same evidence cannot be submitted for both revalidation and appraisal,[39] although care must be taken to ensure that the same evidence can be used for the two different purposes. Concern about the linkage of the two processes remains. There are worries about the confidentiality of the process and whether doctors will feel able to discuss issues that really concern them if the discussion is in any way linked to the certificate that allows them to earn their livelihood.

There is anecdotal evidence[40] to suggest that appraisal is able to refresh parts of the doctor's professional life that no other process has reached. Whether health issues and self-doubts will be expressed in the way that they have been when doctors perceive the link between appraisal and revalidation as undermining the personal value of appraisal, remains to be seen. It is perhaps inherent on the appraiser to ensure that the link is fully understood, that the formative purpose that is at the heart of appraisal remains alive and well, and that necessary and appropriate links to other processes, such as job planning, are explicit and harmonise with the personal development plan.

The importance of the organisation

The place of appraisal within the individual's personal development has thus far been the focus of our thoughts. There are, however, clear benefits of the process for the wider healthcare community and a necessity to ensure that the appraisal process informs the direction of educational provision at a local and national level.

There may, for instance, be local service needs which the appraisee should consider during appraisal in order to decide whether they are able and willing to contribute to their development. For example, a consultant in orthopaedic surgery may be advised during appraisal of a need to develop, in collaboration with elderly care, a shared approach to active management of fractured neck of femur, and may be willing to rise to that challenge. Similarly, a GP may respond to a need to develop unified elderly care or dermatology services across the primary and secondary care interface. In either case, the personal development plan can reflect that new agenda.

The Form 4s that summarise the appraisal discussion, and the personal development plans that accompany them, hold information that is invaluable to the organisation. It is important for the organisation to know if a need for development in a particular area (for example leadership skills) or a particular training need (for example intermediate life support) is identified by several individuals. These should inform the risk management strategy and enable the organisation to consider how to commission educational provision to address common needs.

For doctors who work in less-managed environments there is still a need to ensure that tutors, and other medical educators organising educational programmes, are aware of the needs of local doctors and that the curriculum that is developed is relevant to these learners.

It is not purely in educational matters that a synthesis of the appraisal information is important. There may be organisational issues that impede attendance at educational events (for example the difficulty in obtaining locum cover) or concerns about important areas that may prejudice patient care. The appraisal discussion may highlight areas of poor organisational practice that the individual doctor may feel they cannot otherwise easily take up, especially within the environment of acute trusts. The appraisal should not be a tool to undermine colleagues or criticise organisations, but may allow common themes to be highlighted and addressed.

How can the anonymised forms be used to inform these processes? The appraisal lead should summarise the forms and use the collated findings to produce an annual report,[41] which should be submitted to, and acted upon by, the acute or primary care trust's (PCT) board. There needs to be absolute trust in the confidentiality of the appraisal process and the way in which information is anonymised. An effective process can give a significant strategic steer to NHS organisations and give educational providers, and commissioners of education, a clear direction in curriculum planning.[42]

The same principle applies in a smaller team. Particularly pertinent in primary care (but arguably just as important to teams working together within larger organisations), the sharing of learning needs by individuals within the team enables that team to consider and prioritise learning, allowing the effective use of time and resources.

Clearly there will be personal learning needs, which are personal and should remain so. However, if two doctors in a team identify a need to attend a course in critical reading, for example, one might attend and the other might learn (almost) as much from discussing the issues with the doctor who attended. The sharing of learning with colleagues is important and also serves to focus the 'primary learner' on the main issues raised at a conference or lecture to share with 'secondary learners'.

This principle is taken one step further in practice professional development plans (PPDPs),[43,44] where the individuals' learning needs are used to stimulate a group's development, taking into consideration the other pressures on and needs of the group as a whole.

The challenge

The appraiser meets the appraisee for the annual appraisal discussion. They use that time to help doctors reflect on their professional practice and plan their continuing professional development. This calls for practical and organisational skills that are dealt with elsewhere in this book. The appraiser, as well as sharing a mutual understanding with the appraisee of the purpose of appraisal, needs to consider the wider picture. The way doctors learn, their individual motivations and how they fit into the organisation's development needs to be a thread that runs through the whole appraisal.

An understanding of the principles that underpin appraisal will equip appraisers to support appraisees in considering and refining their professionalism.

References

1 Grant J, Chambers E and Jackson G. *The Good CPD Guide: a practical guide to managed CPD.* Sutton: The Joint Centre for Education in Medicine; 1999.
2 Kolb DA. *Experiential Learning: experience as the source of learning and development.* Englewood Cliffs, NJ: Prentice Hall; 1984.
3 Rogers C, Freiburg HJ. *Freedom to Learn.* Upper Saddle River, NJ: Prentice Hall; 1994.
4 Peyton JWR. *Teaching and Learning in Medical Practice.* Rickmansworth: Manticore Press; 1998.
5 Jarvis P. *Adult and Continuing Education.* New York: Routledge; 1995.
6 Maslow A. Defence and growth. In: Silberman ML, editor. *The Psychology of Open Teaching and Learning.* Boston, MA: Little Brown; 1972. pp. 43–51.
7 Howell W, Fleishman E. *Human Performance and Productivity (Volume 2). Information processing and decision making.* Hillsdale, NJ: Erlbaum; 1982.
8 Luft J. *Group Processes: an introduction to group dynamics.* 2nd ed. Palo Alto, CA: National Press Books; 1970.
9 Conlon M. Appraisal: the catalyst to personal development. *BMJ.* 2002; **327**: 389–91.
10 Houghton A. The whole job type, and how it relates to job satisfaction. *BMJ Careers.* 2004; **329**: 241–2.
11 Quenk N. *Essentials of Myers-Briggs Type Indicator Assessment.* New York: John Wiley and Sons; 2000.
12 Honey P, Mumford A. *The Learning Styles Questionnaire.* Maidenhead: Peter Honey Publication; 2000.
13 Stahl S. Different strokes for different folks: a critique of learning styles. *Am Educ.* 1999; Fall: 1–6.
14 Department of Health. *NHS Appraisal: guidance on appraisal for general practitioners working in the NHS.* London: DoH; 2002.
15 Department of Health. *NHS Appraisal: appraisal for consultants working in the NHS.* London: DoH; 1999.
16 NHS Education Scotland. *GP Appraisal Scheme: a brief guide.* Edinburgh: NHS Scotland; 2003.

17 GP Appraisal and CPD Unit. *GP Appraisal in Wales: annual report 2004/2005.* Cardiff: Cardiff University School of Postgraduate Medical and Dental Education; 2005.

18 Challis M. AMEE Medical Education Guide No 19: Personal Learning Plans. *Med Teach.* 2000; **22**: 225–36.

19 French F, Valentine M. The introduction of personal learning plans for GPs in Grampian, Orkney and Shetland. *Educ Gen Pract.* 1999; **10**(1): 45–55.

20 Lewis M, Elwyn G, Wood F. Appraisal of family doctors: an evaluation study. *Br J Gen Pract.* 2003; **53**(491): 454–60.

21 McKinstry B, Peacock H, Shaw J. GP experiences of partner and external peer appraisal: a qualitative study. *Br J Gen Pract.* 2005; **55**: 539–43.

22 Jelley D, Van Zwanenberg T. Peer appraisal in general practice: a descriptive study in the Northern Deanery. *Educ Gen Pract.* 2000; **11**: 281–7.

23 Lyons N. *Does Involvement in an Appraisal Process Assist General Medical Practitioners in Identification of their Educational Needs and Encourage a Change in Educational Activity in Response to those Needs?* Cardiff: School of Postgraduate Medical and Dental Education, University of Wales College of Medicine; 2003.

24 Holm HA. Review: interactive, but not didactic, continuing medical education is effective in changing physician performance. *Evid Based Med.* 2000; **5**(2): 64.

25 Davis DA *et al.* Changing physician performance. A systematic review of the effect of continuing medical education strategies. *JAMA.* 1995; **274**(9): 700–5.

26 Martin D *et al. Appraisal for GPs.* Sheffield: University of Sheffield, School of Health and Related Research (ScHARR); 2001.

27 Martin D, Harrison P, Joesbury H. *Extending Appraisal to All GPs.* Sheffield: University of Sheffield, School of Health and Related Research (ScHARR); 2003.

28 General Medical Council. *Good Medical Practice.* 3rd ed. London: GMC; 2001.

29 Royal College of General Practitioners. *Good Medical Practice for General Practitioners.* London: RCGP; 2002.

30 Department of Health. *Appraisal Forms for NHS Clinical Consultants.* 2001 [accessed 1 April 2006]. Available from: www.dh.gov.uk/assetRoot/04/03/46/24/04034624.doc

31 Department of Health. *Appraisal Forms for GPs.* 2003 [accessed 1 April 2006]. Available from: www.dh.gov.uk/assetRoot/04/03/50/97/04035097.doc

32. Royal College of Physicians. *Doctors in Society: medical professionalism in a changing world.* London: RCP; 2005.

33 Haman H, Irvine S, Jelley D. *The Peer Appraisal Handbook for General Practitioners.* Oxford: Radcliffe Medical Press; 2001.

34 Chambers R *et al. Appraisal for the Apprehensive: a guide for doctors.* Oxford: Radcliffe Medical Press; 2003.

35 Chambers R *et al. The Good Appraisal Toolkit for Primary Care.* Oxford: Radcliffe Medical Press; 2004.

36 Schon D. *The Reflective Practitioner: how professionals think in action.* 2nd ed. Aldershot: Arena; 1991.

37 Gatrell J, White T. *Medical Appraisal, Selection and Revalidation.* London: Royal Society of Medicine; 2001.

38 Chief Medical Officer. *Good Doctors, Safer Patients.* London: DoH; 2006.

39 National Clinical Governance Support Team. *Defining the Evidence for Revalidation – Supporting the Royal College of General Practitioners. Collation of views from the NHS Clinical Governance Support Team Expert Group.* Leicester: NCGST; 2002.

40 Lyons N. *Quality Assurance Standards for GP Appraisal.* Bury: National Association of Primary Care Educators; 2004.

41 Lyons N. How to write an annual appraisal report. In: Lyons N, editor. *ABC of Appraisal.* Bury: National Association of Primary Care Educators; 2004.

42 Richards T. Continuing medical education. *BMJ.* 1998; **316**(7127): 246.

43 Wilcock P, Campion-Smith C, Elston S. *Practice Professional Development Planning: a guide for primary care.* Oxford: Radcliffe Medical Press; 2003.

44 Pitts J *et al.* Practice professional development plans: general practitioners' perspectives on proposed changes in general practice education. *Br J Gen Pract.* 1999; **49**: 959–62.

Chapter 3

The role of the appraiser

> This chapter defines what the appraiser has to do and the roles an appraiser
> fulfils. It deals with the roles that an appraiser should not attempt to fill and
> describes reasons for choosing to become an appraiser.

Introduction

The role of an appraiser is that of a skilled facilitator. All doctors have confidential
one-to-one discussions with their patients and develop consultation skills to
facilitate that encounter. Because the appraisal is also a confidential one-to-one
discussion, this may go some way to explaining why medical appraisal has been so
readily accepted in most areas[1] despite initial apprehension when it was introduced
as a statutory requirement. Doctors become effective appraisers when they draw
on their existing medical communication and consultation skills.[2]

In order to be successful, however, there are other competencies that an
appraiser must have, because there is a great deal more to the appraisal than just
facilitating a confidential discussion. Just as an effective doctor needs the right
knowledge, skills and attitudes to provide high-quality clinical care throughout a
career, so an appraiser needs the right knowledge, skills and attitudes to carry out
an appraisal discussion effectively and ensure that the time spent is of value to the
appraisee.

Because the scope of an appraisal is so broad, there is an opportunity for the
supportive and confidential discussion to run into very personal and intense areas
of the appraisee's life. Handling this sensitively is a challenge for even the most
skilled appraisers. It is essential that the appraisers are very clear about the limits of
the role they are undertaking.

What does the appraiser do?

The appraiser's job is a privileged one that requires considerable preparation and
time. Some of the tasks performed by the skilful appraiser in the course of one
appraisal cycle are summarised below.

Before the appraisal discussion the appraiser:

- develops the necessary competencies to be able to appraise effectively
- may participate in a local matching process for the allocation of appraisees
- is involved in the organisation of the appraisal discussion (although the detail
  may often be delegated to an administrator or secretary)

- reads and understands the pre-appraisal documentation provided by the appraisee (asking for clarification if necessary)
- prepares for the appraisal discussion.

During the appraisal discussion the appraiser:

- creates the appropriate environment
- clarifies the purpose of appraisal
- emphasises the confidential nature of the discussion
- takes responsibility for the timekeeping and structure of appraisal
- identifies the issues and helps the appraisee to prioritise them
- explores the appraisee's strengths
- explores the appraisee's weaknesses
- explores the constraints on the appraisee
- gives feedback
- establishes the appraisee's development and learning needs
- ensures the appraisal discussion is accurately documented
- facilitates the personal development plan (PDP)
- keeps it real.

After the appraisal discussion the appraiser:

- agrees with the appraisee how the completed paperwork will be shared
- reflects on the appraisal that has just taken place (which may include completion of an evaluation form as in the examples in Chapter 12)
- ensures that the appraiser's key competencies are kept up to date.

It is important that training has prepared the appraiser for all of these roles.

The functions of an effective appraiser

It may be useful, in putting the role of an appraiser in context, to break the role down. Some functions will be provided by every appraiser and are core to each appraisal. Some are functions that are usually inappropriate for appraisers to provide.[3]

Possible roles to consider include:

- chair
- facilitator
- anchor
- key
- signpost
- educational supervisor
- teacher
- doctor
- mentor
- counsellor
- coach
- priest
- friend.

In order to clarify which of these roles are appropriate, it is important to look at what is meant by each of these distinct but complementary functions.

The effective appraiser is the chair

Every meeting, even when there are only two people involved, needs chairing. It is clearly a core function of the appraiser to create the right environment for an appraisal, and revisit and reaffirm the ground rules, particularly emphasising the confidential nature of the discussion. The appraiser should also run the meeting: providing structure and timekeeping, ensuring that all appropriate areas of the appraisal documentation are discussed, taking notes if required and summarising at the end.

The effective appraiser is the facilitator

The role of the appraiser was defined initially as that of a skilled facilitator. What is meant by this?

Facilitation, in the context of appraisal, is:

> Helping appraisees think through where they are now, what they want and need in order to develop as professionals, and how to organise themselves to achieve it.

The effective appraiser is the anchor

Facilitation alone does not capture the role of the appraiser. There seems to be another important function in supporting the appraisee. Some doctors are passing through troubled waters and need a storm anchor. Others have unrealistic expectations of themselves and others, and need anchoring in reality. The skilful appraiser is able to act as an anchor for the appraisee's development.

The effective appraiser is the key

Another important element of the role that is not quite captured by the definition of facilitation is that the appraiser acts as a key to unlock the appraisee's potential. Many doctors seem to require permission to tackle some of their professional challenges, and it can be empowering to discuss their proposals with the appraiser.

The effective appraiser is the signpost

An appraiser should have a good working knowledge of local and national structures and resources that an appraisee might use. In certain circumstances, the appraisee might be pointed towards these by the appraiser. In particular, a list of useful phone numbers or websites is included in most 'appraiser packs'. These can be given to appraisees if appropriate.

By acting as a signpost, the appraiser can help appraisees to go away and do the work themselves, but the first step is made easier for them.

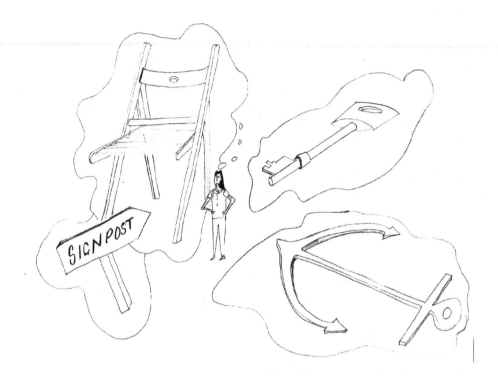

What an effective appraiser is not

Having described what an effective appraiser always is, it is useful to consider which responsibilities an appraiser should not generally take upon themselves.

The appraiser is not the educational supervisor

While some appraisers are drawn from the pool of trained medical educators, many are not. Educational skills in critically reading evidence, giving feedback and knowledge of educational tools can undoubtedly be useful. However, it is not the responsibility of the appraiser to act as the educational supervisor for the appraisee, as the degree of supervision and direction would be inappropriate.

The appraiser is not the teacher

If learning is to be integral to the individual's future professional life, it must be owned by that individual.[4]

Obviously, there may be factual learning needs, particularly about appraisal itself, where the appraiser does 'teach' the appraisee by sharing knowledge and experience. However, the role of teacher does not sit comfortably within appraisal, and the balance should revert back to facilitating the appraisee's reflection as soon as possible.

The appraiser is not the doctor

The overlap between clinical consulting skills and appraisal skills is significant.[5] There may be occasions, particularly when considering health issues, when it is very tempting for appraisers to slip into their more usual role – that of the doctor.

Clinical knowledge may well be used and be useful in the confidential discussion. Appraisers should not forget that they are doctors and therefore have specific skills that can be applied for the benefit of the appraisee. However, it is inappropriate to take medical responsibility for advising an appraisee. Clearly, appraisees with health problems need to be encouraged to seek help first from their own GP, hospital consultant or occupational health service. The appraiser is not there to make medical decisions.

Mentors, counsellors, coaches, priests and friends

Within the appraisal discussion mentoring, counselling and coaching skills may well be applied. However, all of these terms usually imply an ongoing relationship and this is where they differ substantially from the annual appraiser–appraisee relationship.

Some doctors may appear to have a need for ongoing support after the appraisal discussion. It is not appropriate for the appraiser to take on this responsibility. Depending on the particular issues identified, any of the above may be a useful resource and the appraisee might be encouraged at appraisal to consider them as options. For example, finding an appropriate mentor might be a very useful point to explore in the PDP.

The differences between mentors, counsellors, coaches (sometimes called life coaches), priests and friends are subtle but important.

The appraiser is not the mentor

A mentor may be considered as a wise colleague who has experience relevant to the issue for the appraisee. Mentors agree to enter into a more or less formal contract to provide ongoing support and guidance for a defined period, meeting on a regular basis with a specific agenda.[6] Co-mentoring is a variation where both parties agree to meet in a relationship of mutual trust and respect, but the structure of the support provided is quite explicit.[6] The similarities with the appraisal relationship are clear, but the ongoing nature of the support over a defined period is very different.

The appraiser is not the counsellor

A counsellor is a trained professional with particularly well-developed listening skills who will usually meet regularly with the appraisee for a defined period to facilitate the appraisee's self-reflection and help them to move forwards with specific issues. It is usually considered as a therapeutic relationship, which the appraiser is not aiming to provide.

The appraiser is not the coach

A coach has the prime function of challenging the appraisee to get motivated to make changes through reflection and homework activities. Regular reviews may provide the ongoing impetus to the appraisee to meet the targets he has set himself. The appraiser cannot be as directive as the coach would be.

The appraiser is not the priest

A priest may well have mentoring, counselling and coaching skills, but brings a specifically spiritual and religious dimension to the support he provides. Religious advisors usually have a prior and long-term relationship with the appraisee. Even appraisers with strong religious views should be self-aware and not attempt to provide religious support.

The appraiser is not the friend

A friend is supportive on an ongoing basis. It is a relationship based on familiarity and mutual trust but cannot include the degree of structure, rigor or challenge that an appraisal must.

Why become an appraiser?

Individuals may have a wide variety of reasons for becoming an appraiser. For those considering whether it is a career option they would like to pursue, it may be useful to examine their own motivation.

Reasons to become an appraiser

There are many valid reasons for choosing to undertake the challenging but rewarding task of becoming an appraiser. These can be divided into those that are essentially altruistic and those that are more personal.[7]

Altruistic reasons

These include:

- contributing to helping others
- supporting particular professional groups (e.g. sessional or part-time doctors, single-handed clinicians)
- believing in and wishing to promote formative appraisal
- improving the appraisal process locally and nationally
- being able to see the benefits of appraisal done well
- enthusiasm for continuing professional development
- having a lot to give: experience and skills
- sharing ideas
- raising standards of medical professionalism.

More personal reasons

These include:

- career variety
- developing skills that may lead to other career opportunities
- personal challenge
- to learn from others
- curiosity
- peer group support
- financial reward
- to avoid clinical work
- to deal with the perceived threat of appraisal
- to stop 'someone else' from doing it.

All reasons to consider taking on the role are equally valid but it helps to be self-aware about personal motivation in order to ensure that taking on the role is the right career choice. A potential new appraiser should consider the decision to apply for the job carefully because of the degree of responsibility required in taking on this privileged role. It does require a significant commitment in terms of time and effort to do well.

Reflections on being an appraiser

Once appraisers have been in the role for some time and undertaken a number of appraisals, they may be able to express other reasons for becoming and remaining appraisers. Experienced appraisers are often the best advocates for the appraisal process and their insights provide a fascinating view of what appraisals can be like in real life.

Box 3.1 Perceptions about appraisal derived from discussions with experienced appraisees[8]

- Appraisal is a very powerful tool for delivering self-reflection and needs to be delivered with care and skill
- The appraisal process gives appraisees an opportunity to air issues of concern and to demonstrate their insight into their problems and the steps they are taking to ensure that they do not impinge on patient care. It supports them as individuals to identify how to move forward following the appraisal itself
- Many appraisers feel 'very privileged' or 'humbled' by the knowledge, skills and attitudes that appraisees display and feel that they learn a lot from their appraisees
- Some of the good ideas learned during appraisals could, with the permission of the appraisees, be shared at a best practice forum
- Some appraisees are disillusioned and surprised to receive positive feedback about their efforts
- Initial wariness by the appraisee can be transformed into enthusiasm for the process by a successful appraisal

---

- Objectivity, confidentiality and feedback skills are appreciated by the appraisees
- Appraiser support groups are a valuable source of peer support
- Most appraisers feel apprehensive about dealing with difficult appraisals
- A certain percentage of appraisees are under significant strain for a variety of reasons and appraisal can help them to generate an action plan to move forward (reducing the risk of burnout before it leads to poor performance)
- It is unlikely for an appraisal to be the first place where an issue of poor performance is recognised. Adequate training can prepare the appraiser for situations where doctors reveal themselves to be in difficulty and so reduce the stress when it does occur
- The benefits of appraisal are felt by appraisers to be potentially enormous in some cases but difficult to measure and quantify
- Research needs to be done to provide evidence for the complex and beneficial outcomes that appraisers believe occur

Conclusion

The role of the appraiser is highly skilled, varied and interesting. It complements clinical skills and may provide an enhanced awareness of communication skills that are also beneficial to patient care. Appraisers vary in their motivation for becoming an appraiser but are generally agreed that there are many benefits to be gained both personally and professionally from undertaking the role.

References

1 Denney M. Annual appraisal: where have we got to? *Educ Prim Care*. 2005; 16: 697–703.
2 Haman H, Irvine S, Jelley D. *The Peer Appraisal Handbook for General Practitioners*. Oxford: Radcliffe Medical Press; 2001.
3 Chambers R, Tavabie A, Mohanna K, Wakley G. *The Good Appraisal Toolkit for Primary Care*. Oxford: Radcliffe Medical Press; 2004.
4 Rogers C, Freiburg HJ. *Freedom to Learn*. Upper Saddle River: Prentice Hall, NJ; 1994.
5 Chambers R, Wakley G, Field S, Ellis S. *Appraisal for the Apprehensive: a guide for doctors*. Oxford: Radcliffe Medical Press; 2003.
6 Bayley H, Chambers R, Donovan C. *The Good Mentoring Toolkit for Healthcare*. Oxford: Radcliffe Medical Press; 2004.
7 Caesar S. *Responses from two cohorts of primary care appraisers*. NAPCE National Conference Report. Bury: NAPCE; 2004.
8 Central Cheshire Primary Care Trust. *GP Appraisal: annual report 2004*. Nantwich: CCPCT; 2004.

Chapter 4

Becoming an appraiser

This chapter guides doctors on their way to becoming effective appraisers and looks at what support they will need to gain those skills. It considers some aspects of the appraisal process, including how to match appraiser and appraisee.

Introduction

All appraisers make the journey from initially contemplating the role to acquiring the skills necessary to be effective. The path through the selection, training and appointment process will be considered in stages. Appraisal systems have to address some particular issues and these will also be discussed.

To become an appraiser, an interested candidate needs first to find out whether there is an opportunity to apply for the post. Reasons why a doctor may choose to become an appraiser have already been considered in Chapter 3.

Differences between the systems in primary and secondary care can be substantial, as can variations between geographical areas, in particular across the four nations of the UK. These inconsistencies will be highlighted where possible.

Once appointed each appraiser should work within a system which provides:

- a structured recruitment and appointment process
- adequate appraiser training
- a matching process for the allocation of appraisees
- ongoing support structures
- quality assurance
- opportunities for continuing professional development as an appraiser.

Recruiting a new appraiser

Recruitment to the role of appraiser varies by place and within different organisations. In secondary care it has often been automatically assumed that clinical directors will undertake this role within their own directorates, or it has been a line management role alongside job planning. In other areas, particularly in primary care, more formal application, selection and interview processes have gradually been adopted.

When the introduction of medical appraisal began in England in 2001, there was a very tight timetable for implementation. Recruitment took place with little consistency in the early stages. Some trusts struggled to meet their commitment to provide an appraisal for all eligible doctors in the first year. This was partly because of delays in selecting and training enough appraisers in the first few months.

By delaying implementation of their systems and paying particular attention to quality assurance from the beginning, Scotland and Wales have rationalised recruitment and training far better than many parts of England.[1,2]

The appraiser's person specification

There was no national guidance available for specifying the characteristics of a suitable appraiser when the appraisal scheme was introduced. Instead, distinct geographical areas became enthused by the idea of 'doing it right' and created their own versions. Where there is some degree of consistency, it was achieved by networking among interested appraisal leads and educators, promoted by groups such as the National Association of Primary Care Educators (NAPCE).[3,4]

In Scotland it was felt that appraisers should be required to have a clinical commitment of at least two clinical sessions per week in order to be eligible for selection as an appraiser.[1]

It seems unlikely that ex-consultants who have moved entirely into medico-legal work will command the respect of their peer group for long if they no longer see patients. Similarly, following retirement, any doctor will soon lose credibility with the appraisees. Criteria should be built into the contract with the appraising organisation so that such appraisers can be given reasonable notice to leave. One to two years post-retirement is probably the longest that credibility can normally be sustained. This is an area where lay involvement may bring a sense of perspective to the issue. The critical proviso is that individuals must have local credibility.

Common suggestions have included that the appraiser should have been practising for at least three years,[3] that they should be approved by the local trust board and/or the local medical committee (LMC), and meet the locally agreed person specification.

Advertising for a new appraiser

The recruitment of an appraiser falls under equal opportunities legislation. Against the person specification, all candidates should have an equal chance of being appointed. This should be irrespective of sex, colour or creed, whether they are full or part time, a consultant or a staff-grade doctor, a GP principal or doing sessional work. The opportunity to apply must be equally available to all who can command the confidence of their appraisees and are able, after training, to demonstrate the necessary competencies. It is essential that recruitment processes are transparent and open. It is therefore important to advertise appropriately.

Many areas have elected to advertise by writing and emailing to all qualifying doctors working in the target population every time there has been a recruitment round for new appraisers. It is also possible to use local newspapers, newsletters, both paper and electronic, bulletin boards and other locally agreed mechanisms.

It has been common practice to restrict the advertising to those practitioners who have been working in an area for a minimum required number of years, and not to advertise nationally. Guidelines on best practice have been developed.[4] One advantage is that local candidates are likely to meet the requirement to command the respect of their peers. They will be approved by their local trust, medical directors, professional executive committee and/or LMC. More importantly, they will usually be part of the local process as appraisees themselves, which will enhance their credibility. However, as appraisal systems develop, appraisal leads and their organisations may have to consider advertising nationally in order not to discriminate against candidates from further away.

It is inappropriate to recruit only by word of mouth, although it may well be the case that a potential candidate is alerted to the adverts by colleagues. The inherent nepotism in any system that does not allow an advert to reach all eligible practitioners is unacceptable. This contrasts with early experiences in primary care where perhaps the majority of appraisers were recruited by personal contact.

Recruitment of appraisers is significantly different in secondary care, but it is just as important for appraisal skills to be considered when appointing to any role that includes appraisal in the job description. Undertaking appraisals may not occupy the biggest portion of a director's time, but it is a process that will influence all development, both individual and corporate, within a directorate. In the same way, the outcomes of appraisal, if used well, can influence all development in primary care.

There is significant potential for existing appraisers to inspire potential candidates to apply for the role. The policy for dealing with ad hoc enquiries about becoming an appraiser, arising after the appraisal discussion, must reflect the needs of the local appraisal team and appraisees. It may be that putting an expression of interest on file to be considered at the next recruitment round is an appropriate response.

If numbers of appraisers are low, then fast-tracking suitable candidates through a selection and training process may be very helpful to the organisation, but it must not be done at the expense of openness and transparency.

Interviewing for a new appraiser

There are clear guidelines about the constituents of an appraisal interview panel in primary care.[4] They state that it should normally include the clinical governance lead and the chief executive of the PCT. In practice, this is rarely the case, as the job is delegated to the appraisal lead and support team, which may include LMC representation.

In future, it seems likely that lay involvement in the interview and selection process will become more important, and possibly mandatory. How to introduce it in a way that adds value to the process for both the public and the profession is still unclear. Trained lay assessors are now used in primary care for all Quality and Outcome Framework (QuOF) assessment visits under the new General Medical Services (GMS) contract. Similar skills may be required to understand the complexities of the appraisal process and to contribute to it. There may thus be a requirement to provide training courses to enable lay individuals to better appreciate the complexities of the appraisal process. These could be run generically across primary and secondary care.

Lay input brings a breadth of perspective to the appointment process that it might otherwise lack. It may also enhance the credibility of the appraisers in the eyes of the public if they have been appointed with lay involvement.

A potential new appraiser should be considered, at interview, against the agreed person specification. Those found to be unsuitable or to lack sufficient experience or credibility should not be appointed. If there are minor concerns about a candidate, but not sufficient to bar them at interview from becoming an appraiser, then it is reasonable to allow them to progress to the training stage, as this provides a further opportunity to assess suitability for the role. It must be made clear to all candidates that training is a key part of the selection process.

Training a new appraiser

In secondary care, because appraisal was considered a core function of some director-level roles, it has not always attracted adequate training or support. However, it is possible for specific appraiser training to be included in the curriculum for the induction of new clinical directors.

There should be a nationally approved core curriculum for new appraiser training, as there is in Scotland and Wales. Although lacking in the past, significant work is going on in this area. An appraiser should expect training in certain basic areas of the appraisal process common to all. An appropriate curriculum will be explored in more detail in Chapter 5.

Appraiser training should include a chance to rehearse the skills required and support the development of the confidence to undertake the first full-length appraisal. There might also usefully be consideration of any local policy variations. A training course should therefore include a discussion of the local appraisal policy document and any appraiser pack that is in use. National courses must be careful not to overlook this aspect of training.

New appraisers and their potential employers need to understand that being accepted for training at interview is not equivalent to being appointed. There is evidence from Scotland that some candidates may fail to demonstrate the knowledge, skills or attitudes required to become a successful appraiser.[5] There is good evidence from outside medicine that a 'bad appraisal' is worse than no appraisal at all.[6]

In Scotland, following training, some prospective appraisers have decided that the role is not for them. However, the data showed that about 92% of individuals undertaking the training in Scotland went on to take up positions. Even those who chose not to become appraisers took from the training a better understanding of the appraisal process, which provides continuing benefit for them in their role as appraisees.

Appointing a new appraiser to the post

At the end of an interview and training process that has resulted in a demonstration of all the necessary competencies, appraisers can expect to be offered a contract which details the specifics of their role and any local agreements. In England, secondary care appraisal has been left within the hospital trusts and often added to individuals' job plans without any specific contractual amendment. In primary care, contracts have been locally derived and vary considerably in pay and conditions. An example is included in Chapter 12.

The quality assurance of the appraiser selection, training and appointment will be discussed in more detail in Chapter 10.

The support of early appraisals

New appraisers will be expected, as part of the training, to undertake their first full-length appraisal in a supported way. This has resource implications for the potential employer.

Various models for supporting this first appraisal have been considered, and implemented successfully, with the permission of both appraiser and appraisee, including:

- having an experienced appraiser sitting in on the whole appraisal
- videoing the appraisal and debriefing afterwards[7]
- discussing the appraisal with the appraisal trainer or a senior appraiser afterwards (in terms of process not confidential content).

These obviously involve different levels of impact on the interview process, with some being more intrusive than others. It might be inhibitory to an appraisee to reveal something important which made them feel vulnerable if the appraisal was being videoed or had an additional appraiser present as an observer. For this reason the first supported appraisal must be handled carefully with appropriate safeguards. Allowing new appraisers to appraise each other first has been found to be a useful exercise.[8]

The supported first appraisal can count as the appraisee's statutory appraisal for the year, if both parties agree. Depending on the situation, the appraisee may choose to have a second formal appraisal with a more experienced appraiser. Sometimes someone who has already been appraised within the year will volunteer to help the new appraiser by having a second appraisal.

Supporting 'solo' appraisals

The first solo appraisals an appraiser undertakes will naturally be more stressful than those that come later when the appraiser is more experienced. It is therefore considered best practice to provide an increased level of support for newer appraisers, with one recommendation being that this extends to the first three appraisals.[3] The exact support required may well vary considerably from individual to individual. A minimum requirement could be that the appraisal lead is available on the day of the appraisal to debrief the appraiser about any issues that might have arisen, with variations including:

- a more formalised debriefing interview structure
- reflective notes completed by the appraiser
- requesting a more detailed level of feedback from the appraisee.

Ongoing support for appraisers

Throughout an appraiser's career, it will be important that they have clear channels of communication and support for any areas of concern. The first point

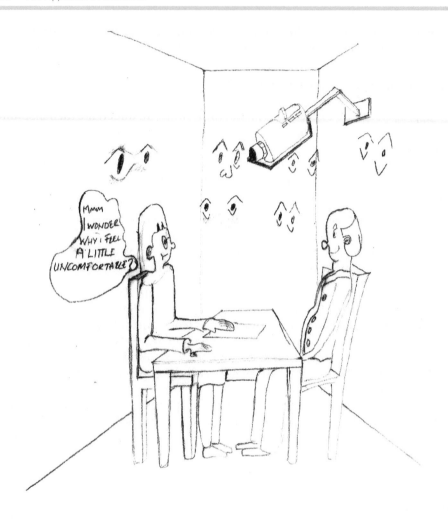

of support might be a 'buddy' within an appraiser support group, or the appraisal lead. It should be clear to all involved what system is in place.

In addition, new appraisers (and their more experienced counterparts) will be concerned with their ability to keep up to date with changes in local and national guidelines, with the ongoing maintenance and enhancement of their skills, and with having a support network of peers.

Appraiser support groups

In many areas of the UK, it has been the experience that local appraisers' support groups have provided an invaluable resource for dealing with appraisers' issues. In particular, they have been used for discussion relating to policies, pay and conditions, the sharing of experiences, discussing difficult appraisals and learning how to manage them better, and working on skills improvements. Functions covered by many appraiser support groups are listed in Box 4.1.

Box 4.1 Roles of appraiser support groups

- Networking and peer support
- Developing communication skills
  - Establishing good rapport
  - Active listening
  - Asking appropriate questions
  - Giving effective feedback
  - Raising sensitive issues
  - Challenging safely
  - Getting back onto safe ground
- Organisational skills
- Facilitating better Form 4s and PDPs
- Dealing with difficult appraisal scenarios
- Learning about educational tools
- Creating the appraiser's resource pack
- Appraisee support
- Housekeeping issues, e.g. pay and conditions

It would appear that in secondary care, there are fewer such groups because individuals have regarded the role more as part of the 'day job', not as one they have chosen to pursue and in which to seek further training.

A support group should not be too large. A group of 50 is too big to develop an action learning set model of development.[9] It should have a reasonable membership, either based on geography or on the number of appraisees within the same system. It does not seem sensible for one hospital trust or one PCT to exclude a handful of members on the grounds that the ideal group size is between eight and 12 when there are, for example, 15 appraisers covering the local clinicians. All individuals should have the opportunity to contribute and be heard, as well as be able to attend.

It seems that in primary care many appraiser support groups operate on a two-tier model. There may be shorter lunchtime or half-day review meetings on a regular basis, bimonthly or quarterly, with annual skills update days when more formal training may be undertaken.

The shorter meetings need to be sufficiently local for all the members of the group to be reasonably able to attend, and the timing of these meetings needs to allow for travel. It may make sense for localities or trusts to pool resources and organise annual skills updates over larger groups and a bigger geographical area, as it is not unreasonable to expect people to travel further for a whole day. There are benefits to be gained from the wider networking that sharing with other local groups allows. It may be helpful to mix appraisers from primary and secondary care in the future.

It is also appropriate for key personnel or lead appraisers from various localities to attend regional or national support events with the aim of sharing best practice and achieving greater national consistency.

A successful appraiser support group should encourage the development of the appraisers as individuals as well as the appraisal process as a whole. The appraisers may need to do some work to support local appraisees, e.g. in developing an appraisee support pack. This group may well also be the appropriate forum to inform appraisees about the requirements of revalidation when they become clear.

Appraisals happen in a potentially intense and isolated environment. It is vital that appraisers have networks of support to counteract this. Benchmarking an individual's practice against that of the peer group is a very powerful learning tool.[10]

Matching of appraiser and appraisee

Every organisation needs to have a system to match appraisees and appraisers. The number of appraisals undertaken by one appraiser within a year can vary widely (one informal survey demonstrated a range from as few as three to as many as 70 in one year).[11] Similarly, clinical directorates in secondary care can vary widely in size, and, if no protected time is allocated for appraisals, having a large number of appraisees can be a considerable burden on the clinical directors, alongside their other roles. Because of this, new models of allocating appraisers to appraisees may need to be considered for secondary care as well.

Three basic models are considered below.

- Dual veto systems.
- Choice option systems.
- Allocation systems (both straightforward and special allocations).

In a dual veto system, all appraisees are given a list of all available appraisers and invited to veto all those with whom they think they could not have a satisfactory appraisal, and the appraisers have an equal opportunity to veto appraisees. They are not required to give a reason but the veto is absolute, and a random allocation process takes place subsequently taking into account the vetoes expressed.

In a choice option system, the appraisee is allocated a small number of appraisers and asked to choose between them.

Straightforward allocations occur when there is no element of choice or veto prior to the matching process. Once matched, however, either the appraiser or the appraisee can ask for one alternative if the first match is unacceptable to them, and this would normally be granted except in exceptional circumstances.

Special allocations occur when an appraiser with particular skills is chosen deliberately for a particular appraisee. Sometimes this relates to the requirements for a joint appraisal (Chapter 9) or to a particular issue for the appraisee.

Are vetoes dangerous or a possible management tool?

Concerns have been voiced that it may be threatening to the appraisers to be vetoed by the appraisees. In one matching, in primary care, every possible appraiser had at least two vetoes. It was therefore a very levelling process.[12]

Despite being told specifically that they did not have to give a reason, most of the vetoes expressed by appraisees were explained by one of the following:

- patient
- close colleague, e.g. GP partner

- spouse
- friend
- own GP.

Doctors seemed to feel a need to explain their reason when they vetoed someone they liked. No explanation may have indicated a personal dislike. There was no evidence of systematic vetoes for gender, geography, or being a full- or part-time doctor. Because most of the vetoes were explained and were for positive reasons, using the number of vetoes against a particular appraiser prior to appraisal as a performance management measure would be inappropriate.[13]

Matching for appraisers

Because of the particular networking and discussion that a local appraiser support group provides, it is clear that members of the same group cannot continue to appraise each other for long. This would appear collusive. In many areas, this concern has led to systems for cross-border appraisals, where members of neighbouring appraiser support groups agree to appraise one another. These reciprocal arrangements can be very effective.

How often should the appraiser change?

There is a great deal of discussion among appraisers about the differences between first and second appraisals with the same appraisee. So much of the relationship building has often already happened during the first appraisal that there may be a chance to make the second more focused and a good opportunity to challenge the appraisees to stretch themselves a little further. If an appraisee has really moved forwards throughout the year, the praise and support of the appraiser will be particularly apt and meaningful.

But what if an element of collusion has arisen? What if the matching is not really giving a satisfactory working relationship? What if the appraisee has learned all he can from this particular appraiser?

Although some appraisers feel strongly that no more than three consecutive appraisals should be undertaken by the same appraiser–appraisee pairing, national quality assurance guidelines suggest that a change every two years is wiser.[4] This would allow for three different appraisers in every five-year revalidation cycle, surely enough to avoid the possibility that the appraisal might be considered simply a 'cosy chat'.

By contrast, in secondary care, appraisees may never have the opportunity to change their appraiser under current systems and this may be seen as a risk. It needs to be acknowledged and addressed as secondary care appraisal systems develop.

How long should an appraisal take?

The time taken for an individual appraisal has been very variable. It depends in part on the commitment of the commissioning body, e.g. PCT or hospital trust, to the process. Some in primary care have been given a full 3.5-hour session. The exact timing then depends on the response of the appraiser and appraisee to the appraisal. In one informal survey, the range of time taken for the full appraisal discussion, including the completion of all the relevant paperwork, varied from two to five hours.[12] There are, however, anecdotal accounts of appraisals lasting as little as an hour.

> 'I had spent quite some time preparing for my appraisal and to have a discussion that only lasted an hour, with coffee time included, felt like a slap in the face.'

This might indicate a lack of commitment or a very collusive attitude and would certainly need to be subject to scrutiny in any quality assurance process. There may be a probity issue if the appraiser is being paid for the full 3.5-hour session. If the recommendation to complete the paperwork there and then cannot be met, it is the total time taken that should be considered, not just the time spent on the appraisal discussion.

Appraising the appraisal role

The role of the appraiser has been described in Chapter 3. Although it is possible to include appraising this role, under 'Teaching and training' in Form 3 of the standard appraisal paperwork, it is sometimes considered in its own right.

One useful resource is a version of the teaching and training page of the appraisal documentation adapted for appraisal. This can be used whether the discussion is within the main clinical appraisal, or a separate appraisal process, usually facilitated by the appraisal lead.

A separate appraisers' appraisal?

The appraisal lead may set up an annual one-to-one confidential meeting with each appraiser. During this discussion, strengths, weaknesses and areas of constraint may be identified, to build into the PDP for the individual, or the following year's appraiser support group learning objectives or action plan. The appraiser should be given the individual feedback from the post-appraisal evaluation forms arising from the appraisals he has undertaken. This is also a great opportunity to feed back to the organisation about any problems with the appraisal systems locally.

If it is run separately, the outcomes can be included in the clinical appraisal documentation under the section for 'others who have contributed to this process'.

This is an appraisee-led formative process. There may also be a requirement for a separate performance management review.

Conclusion

An appraiser requires advanced skills, particularly communication skills, to perform well in this privileged role. Candidates must, therefore, demonstrate the required competencies and pass a summative process of selection and training in order to be appointed. They need particular support with the first few appraisals that they undertake and an ongoing network of peer support to deal with the issues that can arise. The organisation has a responsibility for establishing a quality-assured system within which they can work effectively.

Appraisers need to be appraised specifically in their appraisal role. They need feedback from their appraisees and must be committed to continual professional development as appraisers.

References

1 NHS Education Scotland. *GP Appraisal Scheme: a brief guide*. Edinburgh: NHS Scotland; 2003.
2 GP Appraisal and CPD Unit. *GP Appraisal in Wales: annual report 2004/2005*. Cardiff: Cardiff University School of Postgraduate Medical and Dental Education; 2005.
3 Lyons N. *Quality Assurance Standards for GP Appraisal*. Bury: National Association of Primary Care Educators; 2004.
4 National Clinical Governance Support Team. *Assuring the Quality of Medical Appraisal: report of the NHS Clinical Governance Support Team Expert Group*. Leicester: NCGST; 2005.
5 Murie J. GP appraisal recruitment in Scotland 2005. *BMJ Career Focus*. 2005; **331**(7512): gp59–60.
6 Murphy K, Cleveland J. *Understanding Performance Appraisal*. London: Sage; 1995.
7 Mohanna K. *Appraiser Self-assessment Communication Skills Workbook*. London: Royal College of General Practitioners; 2005.
8 Essex Appraisal Steering Group. *GP Appraisal in Essex: the Essex scheme*. Chelmsford: Essex Appraisal Steering Group; 2002.
9 Jacques D. *Learning in Groups*. 3rd ed. London: Kogan Page; 2000.
10 Chambers R, Mohanna K, Wakley G, Wall DW. *Demonstrating Your Competence 1: healthcare teaching*. Oxford: Radcliffe Medical Press; 2004.
11 National Association of Primary Care Educators. *Pay and Conditions Questionnaire*. National Appraisal Conference 2004. Market Bosworth: NAPCE; 2004.
12 Central Cheshire Primary Care Trust. *GP Appraisal: annual report 2004*. Nantwich: CCPCT; 2004.
13 Caesar S. *Some Lessons from Appraiser–Appraisee Matching*. National Appraisal Conference 2004. Market Bosworth: NAPCE; 2004.

Chapter 5

The appraiser training curriculum

This chapter sets out a curriculum for appraiser training, based on the key competencies demonstrated by skilful appraisers. It includes some common appraiser and appraisee pitfalls that all appraisers should be aware of.

Introduction

There is a need to define a curriculum for appraiser training. In the past, the effects of geography and luck have played an inappropriately significant part in the training of individual appraisers. Only a few areas have had clearly defined agendas for appraiser training.[1]

There has been some work on defining core competencies for appraisers.[2] Appraisal training providers have often created their own checklist of core skills to be taught. As a result, the first national guidance for England has been published.[3]

Appraiser training in primary and secondary care should have a consistent core curriculum. Such training is an ongoing requirement, both in terms of learning new skills and revisiting and honing existing ones, especially given the evolving nature of appraisal and the context of a rapidly changing NHS. A syllabus simply includes the what and the why, of competencies being taught,[4] but the curriculum will also address the how and the when.

In its broader sense, the curriculum encompasses educational content, aims and outcomes, strategy and delivery. Training providers will need to think about the content of the curriculum and remember that learning occurs both in the 'taught' curriculum and informally between participants. It is important to think about how to encourage learning outside teaching.

Appraisers should be required to demonstrate key competencies in their knowledge, skills and attitudes. The evaluation of their success or failure to do so should be transparent and fair. The purpose of appraiser training should be to improve the individual's capabilities with instruction, practice and honest feedback. By the end of new appraiser training, only those who are able to demonstrate the required standards in all areas being assessed should be recommended for appointment.

The medical appraiser's curriculum

The syllabus

Knowledge

- The scope and purpose of appraisal and revalidation, and how it compares with assessment and performance management.
- The requirements of the appraisal process, including local, regional and national variations where relevant.
- The environment within which the appraisee is practising.
- The rules of confidentiality.
- The duties and responsibilities of doctors.[5,6]
- Procedures regarding poor performance as they relate to appraisal.
- How to access occupational health resources.
- Grounds for stopping an appraisal.

Skills

- Organisational skills, including setting up the appraisal, preparing the pre-appraisal paperwork and dealing promptly with any queries.
- Information technology (IT) skills, including an ability to use electronic appraisal systems such as the NHS Toolkit/Welsh online system.[7]

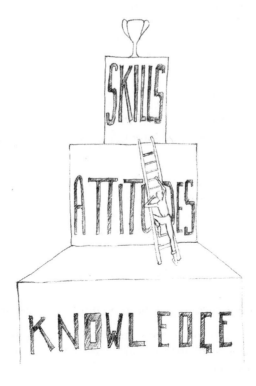

- Evaluation skills, including the critical assessment of a portfolio of evidence.
- Chairmanship skills, including creating the right environment for the appraisal and guiding the appraisal process.
- Communication skills, including active listening, open questioning and feedback skills, challenging effectively and getting back to safe ground.
- Educational skills, including a toolbox of possible needs assessment resources and an awareness of different learning styles.
- Paperwork facilitation skills, including writing a good Form 4 and developing a useful personal development plan (PDP).
- Skills in dealing with difficult appraisals.

Attitudes

- Self-aware.
- Free from bias and prejudice.
- Non-judgemental.
- Constructively challenging.
- Supportive and understanding.
- Professional.

Ground rules for appraiser training

'Ground rules' are a set of commonly owned principles by which all the individuals in a small group agree to abide. They define the expectations of group members towards one another within the context of the team. Agreeing the ground rules forms a very important part of building the shared trust and confidence that allows effective work in small groups.[8] At the very outset of training it is important to clarify the 'ground rules' to be applied (*see* Chapter 11).

Although every group will define its own rules, common starting points are laid out in Box 5.1.

Box 5.1 Ground rules for small group work
- Confidentiality – agreeing a shared definition of confidentiality for the group
- Respect
- Honesty
- Constructive comments
- Listening
- No interruptions, including switching off mobiles
- Punctuality

The appraiser training curriculum: how it should be taught

Having done some basic introductions and work on establishing ground rules, appraiser training will be ready to move on to the specific areas that need covering. The personal preferences and teaching styles of different providers will have a large impact on the techniques used. There are many effective models for training, which differ substantially in design. However, introducing the candidates to the core competencies they need to demonstrate will be common to all training approaches. It is worth breaking down the curriculum for all appraisers and considering key issues here.

Training new appraisers: knowledge

The scope and purpose of appraisal

Although this is covered in more depth in Chapter 1, it is useful to consider the similarities and differences between appraisal and revalidation (Table 5.1) and assessment and performance management (Table 5.2). With a thorough understanding of these in the context of medical appraisal, the scope and purpose of appraisal becomes clear. It is a useful first exercise to get potential appraisers to explore their preconceptions about these differing but complementary processes.

The appraisal process

Appraiser training should include an understanding of the local, regional and national appraisal processes. A timetable for the general process is described in Chapter 6. It is desirable for every area to produce an appraiser's pack with useful local contacts and guidelines. Training should include a discussion about the contents of the local pack. A suggested content list for 'The Appraiser Pack' is included in Chapter 6.

In those areas where such a pack does not exist, training should include information about those resources that every appraiser will want. In this way a local or regional pack will rapidly be developed. In addition, there are examples of

Table 5.1 Appraisal and revalidation: definitions and differences

Appraisal	Revalidation
Formative	Summative
NOT pass/fail	IS Pass/Fail
Confidential	Public
Statutory	Statutory
Internal accountability	External accountability
Supportive	NOT supportive
Reflective	NOT reflective
Educational	NOT educational
Facilitated self-assessment of development needs	Demonstration of continuing fitness for practice
Results in personal development plan	Results in licence to practice

Table 5.2 Assessment and performance management: definitions and differences

Assessment	Performance management
Measurement	Measurement
Usually summative but can be formative	Summative
Judgemental Comparative Analytical	Judgemental Comparative
Can identify learning needs	May be linked to rewards or sanctions
Set against predetermined standards (internal or external)	Set against external standards

Table 5.3 Issues facing the appraisee

Generic	Individual
Cultural Educational Occupational Environmental	Nature of employment Stage of career Family commitments Other roles and commitments

useful resources held electronically on some of the national Web-based resources, e.g. www.appraisalsupport.nhs.uk and www.napce.net. Best practice can then be shared and duplication of effort minimised.

The environment in which the appraisee practises

Although all doctors are appraisees, they practise in differing environments. The appraiser needs to be aware of the issues facing an individual appraisee. Some of the contextual factors are considered in Table 5.3. For example, in a clinic where a large proportion of patients are immigrants or refugees, a multitude of different languages will be spoken. Getting adequate interpreter support can be a major difficulty, and confidentiality and chaperones can pose particular challenges.

Training on confidentiality

There is a great risk in making presumptions that all doctors share the same understanding about what constitutes a breach of confidence. In terms of new appraiser training, there are two aspects that particularly need to be revisited.

Confidentiality within appraisal

To create the trust required for appraisal, both parties must share the same understanding of confidentiality. It is vital at the start of every appraisal to spell out the ground rules for the appraisal with the appraisee. There is a risk of derailing a very important level of disclosure later, if appraisees are not made aware, in advance, of circumstances in which an appraisal would need to be stopped. Situations where the appraisal has been used as a 'cry for help' are fortunately very rare.

The responses that can be made to a first disclosure of poor performance, serious illness or whistle blowing will be dealt with in more detail later in this chapter.

Confidentiality within appraiser support groups

There is always a risk in appraisers discussing problems they have encountered which the appraisee would feel to be a breach of confidentiality of the appraisal. It is therefore imperative that a training or support group has explicit ground rules about what is and is not reasonable to discuss. Most scenarios can be successfully made anonymous. If they could not, and the identity of the appraisee would be revealed by the detail of the discussion, then it should not be brought to the appraiser support group in that form. Major issues should be dealt with one to one with the appraisal or clinical governance lead according to local policy.

The risk of Barnum statements

Barnum statements, named after the famous American showman Phineas Taylor Barnum (1810–1891), are widely used by fortune tellers and clairvoyants. They are defined as:

> Non-specific statements designed to engage as many people as possible on an individual level (by sounding specific).

Appraisers need to be aware of them because:

- people are inevitably very sensitive to Barnum statements
- we must be aware of the need for confidentiality at all times.

I tried to enliven a talk about appraisal with examples that my audience could relate to, and used two fictitious examples:

> '. . . appraisal is a powerful process because it can support people with all sorts of issues, from a junior partner who felt that all her ideas were being stifled by an unsupportive senior partner, to someone who, through discussing the death of his father many years before, was able to deal with some issues of loss and grief.'

However, two people in the audience thought that I was talking specifically about someone they knew.

This is particularly important for appraisal support groups. If, in discussion, a case is made anonymous by, for example, changing the sex of an appraisee and the substance of addiction, and talking about the disclosure of Ritalin abuse by a female GP, there will (probably) be someone out there who is that GP, even though the experience may actually have been with a male Methadone abuser.

The duties and responsibilities of doctors

It is imperative that every appraiser is familiar with the guidance laid out in the documents *Good Medical Practice*[5] and *Good Medical Practice for General Practitioners*[6] (for GPs). Any potential appraiser who is not sufficiently motivated or organised to be able to read these before undertaking training has not demonstrated the necessary attitudes to become an effective appraiser. Without this knowledge, no discussion of the areas of good medical practice, including health or probity issues in particular, can be satisfactorily undertaken.

Poor performance procedures

Every area should have a very clearly defined structure for dealing with poor performance issues. This usually involves a poor performance panel, which assesses an individual situation and decides on the appropriate response. Options to resolve a performance issue may be: local, involve the National Clinical Assessment Service (NCAS), now part of the National Patient Safety Agency (NPSA), or include referral to the General Medical Council (GMC).[9]

Appraisers need to know how to stop the appraisal and be aware of how to access this process, but not necessarily all the intricacies of dealing with poor performance from start to finish.

Occupational health resources

From time to time, it is likely that most appraisers will come across appraisees who have significant health issues. If these put patients at risk, then the appraisal should be stopped. Such situations will be discussed in more detail in Chapter 9. More often, the appraisal will be able to be completed satisfactorily, but the appraiser may need to point appraisees in the direction of local occupational health resources, their own GP or a consultant. An up-to-date knowledge of these resources by the appraiser is therefore important.

The limits of the appraisal process

When and how to stop an appraisal that has moved into the territory of whistle blowing, illness, poor performance or any type of crisis is a subject that terrifies most new appraisers. It is worth spending considerable time on building confidence in the appraiser's ability to recognise such rare situations and practising the skills needed to handle them, even though most appraisers will not need to call on such knowledge and skills. The confidence that comes from having rehearsed potentially difficult scenarios is invaluable.

Training new appraisers: skills

Organisational skills

All appraisers need sufficient organisational skills to handle the detail of the appraisal process, including setting up the appraisal, preparing the pre-appraisal paperwork and dealing promptly with any queries. Appraisal administrators and secretaries may get very frustrated if an appraiser is haphazard and fails to deal properly with the paperwork involved. More important still, the appraisees will not value a process if the appraiser does not seem to respect it. It is rare for these skills to be formally taught and assessed on new appraiser training, but if they cannot be demonstrated by a candidate, it would be fairer to all concerned if the candidate were not appointed.

Someone who is advised that this is the reason for being turned down may have the impetus to make changes to their personal time management or working style and become a suitable candidate at some future point. Disorganisation is often an attitudinal issue about respecting the process, or a lifestyle issue arising from over-commitment.

IT skills

Appraiser training needs to ensure that appraisers have the minimum IT skills required to support appraisees who choose to work electronically. This means they need to be able to navigate, for example, the NHS Toolkit or the Welsh online appraisal documentation.[7,10] They do not need to be computer 'whiz kids', but they do need to be comfortable enough not to try to influence the appraisee against presenting information electronically.

Training must include the specifics of the relevant online systems.

Evaluation skills

The skills required to prepare for an appraisal, including dealing with the paperwork, are covered in more detail in Chapter 6. Appraisers, particularly those who come to appraisal with no formal training in medical education, may be daunted by the idea of reading a portfolio of evidence critically. Adequate training in this area can relieve many anxieties and allow a new appraiser to go to the appraisal confident of being well prepared.

Chairmanship skills

How to achieve the relaxed, open and comfortable environment required for a satisfactory appraisal is dealt with in more detail in Chapter 7. Getting the process right as an organisation, arriving punctually, setting the scene with a suitable introduction and gauging the right manner in which to approach a particular appraisee all have a part to play.

The in-depth knowledge of the local appraisal process will allow the appraiser to take responsibility for managing the timekeeping, paperwork and structure of the appraisal. The ability to both develop and address the appraisal agenda within the allotted time is a significant skill. It is not helpful to be too rigid. The 'best laid plans of mice and men gang aft agley'.[11]

Without a basic structure in mind, however, it is difficult to develop the flexibility to deal with the unexpected.

Communication skills

Communication skills are central to most of what doctors do. They are now taught at all stages of the medical curriculum. There are increasingly few doctors who do not have a formal awareness of them. Communications skills, including active listening, open questioning and feedback skills, challenging effectively and getting back to safe ground will be covered in more detail in Chapter 7. It is appropriate to present them in the context of the appraisal discussion. From the point of view of the curriculum, it is enough to highlight the need for specific training in communication skills in relation to the appraisal process.

Educational skills, including a toolbox of possible resources

An overview of adult learning theory as applied to appraisal has been laid out in Chapter 2, along with a consideration of the importance of learning style preferences in making learning opportunities as effective as possible. New appraiser training will incorporate these ideas into the vocabulary with which the new appraiser is being equipped. In addition, there are other tools that a new appraiser will want to have to hand. Candidates with no previous educational experience, in particular, may not have met some of these tools previously and so may need specific training. They may usefully be directed to suitable resources in which to read about tried-and-tested techniques.[12,13]

There are many different tools available. The nature and importance of the needs they identify is not equivalent. Some directly reflect impact on patient care; others look at insight, or knowledge. A range of methods is therefore needed to best look at performance for the formative purposes of appraisal.

It is important that all appraisers have a clear understanding of how to facilitate the appraisee's personal needs assessment. Without knowing what an appraisee's learning and development needs are, how can the PDP be powerful enough to drive change?

Box 5.2 The needs assessment toolkit
- Identification of PUNs and DENs[14]
- Sticky moments
- Self-assessment tools, including PEP CDs
- Significant event analysis (SEA)
- Complaints
- Random case analysis
- Case-based discussion
- Analysis of referral and prescribing data
- Audit
- Reflective learning logs (reflection in action and reflection on action)
- Electronic tools (*see* Chapter 11)
- NHS Toolkit
- 360-degree appraisal
- Patient feedback

PUNs and DENs

PUNs are 'patients' unmet needs' and DENs are 'doctors' educational needs' (which often, but not always, arise from an awareness of patients unmet needs).[14] This simple but effective tool involves the clinician taking a small amount of time at the end of a patient encounter to reflect on it. Where the doctor becomes aware of something that was on the patient's agenda but was not addressed, it becomes a PUN. It may be that it was entirely appropriate to choose not to address it, but at least it has been brought into the open area of Johari's Window[13] and the doctor is not blind to it. Deciding whether it becomes a DEN and, if so, what to do about it, is the second stage of the reflection. Often all that is required is to look up an area of uncertainty, or a mental note to tackle the 'by the way' comment next time.[14]

Sticky moments

All doctors will recognise the concept of 'sticky moments', when they suddenly become aware of a difficulty in terms of knowledge, skills or attitude. Formalising this into an easily memorable tool for needs assessment has been described[15] and may intuitively appeal to some appraisees.

Self-assessment tools

There are an increasing variety of self-assessment tools available. The advent of revalidation is likely to generate even more. Perhaps the most familiar to doctors are the online e-learning modules (Chapter 11). The great advantage of these is the complete flexibility they provide for clinicians to do them at a time that is convenient. Most tools provide a print-out certificate that details the subject covered and when it was done. One possible disadvantage is that it is rarely clear before starting to use one of these tools how relevant the level of information presented and tested will be. There is not yet a single system for kite-marking tools of this type.

In addition the Royal College of General Practitioners (RCGP) has produced CD ROMs that have been tried and tested particularly with registrars. These Phased Evaluation Project CDs (PEP CDs), the latest CD edition of which is called PEP-QB, may be useful to some appraisees. These CD resources are being superseded by internet-based versions.

Significant event analysis

Significant events are those from which lessons can be learned. They may be positive, when something has been handled particularly well. They may relate to so-called 'near misses' where an individual has become aware of something that could have gone wrong but didn't, or at least didn't cause any significant harm. Of course, sometimes they relate to a negative event, where something was handled badly or something went wrong. Analysis of such awareness can often strengthen systems and teams to capitalise on success or prevent similar negative events occurring in the future.

It is vital that the NHS creates a culture whereby learning from mistakes is seen as natural and essential. Burying mistakes only means that they will recur because the systems and attitudes that allowed them to happen have not been changed.

> Every system is perfectly designed to get the results it gets.
>
> **Don Berwick**

In primary care, the importance of SEA has been emphasised by incorporating the requirement to do at least 12 a year in the QuOF assessment targets. Significant events can be recorded under a traffic light system, with events entered into a file for discussion by any member of the team under a green (positive), amber (near miss, should be learned from) and red (serious negative) code. There may be a temptation only ever to look at the red codes, but actually reminding the appraisee that things do also go well by looking at green can usefully be emphasised by the appraiser.

Complaints

Every doctor dreads receiving a complaint. Unfortunately, in our increasingly litigious society, most doctors can expect to have several complaints made against them during their working life. The public are encouraged to complain as consumers and bring this attitude with them to medicine. The anger and fear that illness and death understandably provoke are a particularly fertile ground for seeking to apportion blame. 'It must be somebody's fault.'

Most complaints are minor and can be handled by appropriate and sensitive in-house systems. Some are mischievous or malicious. A few are more serious. They can be simplistically categorised into those arising from administrative or operational difficulties, and those where there is a suspicion of clinical error or malpractice.

The appraiser can have a vital role in helping an appraisee who has been the subject of a complaint. There is a need for an exploration of the emotions aroused: the feelings of self-doubt, anger and guilt that can arise. The appraiser can also help the doctor to benchmark what occurred to gain a sense of perspective. There may be genuine learning points for the appraisee which need to be considered in the next year's PDP. Unless the potential distress caused by the complaint has been acknowledged and dealt with, little useful learning is likely to be possible. Once the appraiser has facilitated the processing of the emotion, the doctor with a complaint will often highlight the key learning that needs to occur.

Random case analysis

Random case analysis is another simple tool that can be very effective. There are established pro formas that can be used to structure the discussion about a particular case.[15] Alternatively, appraisees may choose to use their own structure. One key feature is that the cases are genuinely chosen at random, e.g. the 'n'th patient in the outpatient clinic. It is a tool that can be used by the appraisee alone as a means to aid reflection or in groups where the cases are discussed.

Case-based discussion

Case-based discussion is structured around cases that have been chosen specifically to highlight some learning point or need. Asking an appraisee to reflect on the most satisfying case they have seen over the past month, and follow up with the least satisfying, with paired questions, is an approach that can be used effectively within appraisal. The cases chosen are no longer random and the learning will therefore be different. As a tool it is useful for disclosing the appraisees' insight into their professional judgement.

Analysis of referral and prescribing data

Referral and prescribing data have been highlighted for analysis because of the significant implications of above-average referral or prescribing behaviour in terms of resources for the NHS, and below-average figures and the implications for patient safety. Most doctors believe that they make judgements on the basis of best practice. Discussion of how and why an appraisee's figures differ from those of their colleagues can lead to powerful insights into the doctor's professional judgement. Comparative data must be accurate and discussion must explore and allow for confounding factors. A doctor who looks after many nursing homes will prescribe more palliative and terminal care medication and have more deaths than one who looks after a student population in a university town. The exploration of differences is one of the most fertile grounds for encouraging individuals to challenge themselves. Of course, it is instinctive for appraisees to defend their decisions, and appraisers have to be skilled in hearing out the defensiveness and allowing the appraisees to move on to the next stage of questioning themselves.

Audit

Many doctors feel that audit is 'not for them'. They are happy for it to be done by other members of the team but find it hard to prioritise this activity within the time constraints that exist and the clinical care they wish to provide. This is less true for surgeons and those whose clinical practice lends itself easily to measurement, who are used to using audit as a tool from their early training onwards. There is likely to be some kind of defined expectation for all clinicians to undertake audit.

The appraiser can have a formative role in helping doctors who are nervous about audit to think of a simple question that they wish to ask about their clinical care and helping them to define an audit for their PDP. Appraisers also have a key role in helping the appraisee to ensure that the audit cycle is completed and the learning incorporated back into practice.

Reflective learning logs

There are a significant proportion of clinicians who are able to use reflective diaries as useful tools. However, there is some evidence that even among motivated higher professional education (HPE) doctors only 70% had the discipline and aptitude to maintain them for a year.[16] It is a tool for the appraisers to use with care so that they do not set up appraisees to fail. However, there is no ducking the issue that reflective practice should be a cornerstone of medical professionalism.[17] The reflective cycle should be a routine and constant part of every doctor's thinking. It is the recording of the evidence for it that seems problematic to many. An appraiser's help can be invaluable in supporting the appraisees in finding systems that will be effective for them. There is no need for an appraisee to be driven to excessive lengths to keep records beyond the minimum required for training purposes or to provide evidence.

Considering 'reflection in action' and 'reflection on action' may be helpful to some appraisees.[18]

Electronic tools

There are a variety of educational electronic tools that can:

- record what the practitioner has reflected upon
- provide information and patient leaflets.

One electronic tool that many GPs find useful is GP Notebook,[19] which can be set up to run in the background to the clinical system that they use and which can record every time the clinician looks something up online. A print-out at the end of the year provides evidence of the types of topic and frequency with which the clinician looks things up. One perceived difficulty with this as a tool is that sometimes the frequency with which something is looked up is not a good measure of learning need. A doctor may never prescribe for a child without checking the children's dose, but this may be evidence of good practice rather than a weakness. Indeed, it can be said that what a modern clinician needs to know is not the details of best practice (which are subject to frequent change) but where to look them up.

In preparing for the appraisal, the appraiser needs to be aware that the certificates produced from these tools are a record of access not of learning. The reflection that goes with them is what either makes them useful to the appraisee, or not.

NHS Toolkit

There is an entirely electronic version of the appraisal documentation developed by the Sowerby Centre for Health Informatics at Newcastle (SCHIN) working with the Department of Health.[7] All appraisers need a working knowledge of how to register and log on to the system. They can then access their appraisee's forms and deal with them online. As more appraisees choose to work electronically and upload their documentation and supporting evidence, so the corresponding need for IT skills in appraisers grows.

The Welsh appraisal system has entirely electronic paperwork and so all Welsh appraisers have specific training needs to use this effectively.

360-degree or multi-source feedback

There are many systems designed to collect feedback from people who are in all types of contact with the subject (the 'goldfish bowl' or 360-degree view). In professional terms, they are often subdivided into groups called 'bosses', 'peers' and 'direct reports'. As long as there are sufficient numbers in each group then the report can be rendered anonymous such that the subject cannot directly attribute comments. This is meant to lead to increased honesty in feedback. Of course, sometimes very useful feedback is not anonymous but delivered in a constructive way by a trusted individual. There are many different multi-source feedback tools on the market. Some may be implemented organisationally rather than individually. The skill lies in facilitating the reflection on the feedback.

Because the methods often use a structured questionnaire, some models suggest that the appraisee completes the questionnaire too, because there are valuable insights to be gained from comparing and contrasting the self-assessment with the feedback form others.

Patient feedback

Our staunchest allies and our sternest critics are likely to be our patients. Patient satisfaction surveys of various types, e.g. CFEP[20] and GPAQ[21], have recently gained widespread use because of the QuOF requirement for GPs in particular to seek to understand what their patients think of the service they provide. Simpler ideas, like suggestions boxes, and other channels of communication have been in place for many years, although they have not always produced any great insights.

The appraiser needs to be able to facilitate the reflection that the appraisee makes on the results of whatever survey they have undertaken. This is much easier when the survey is produced to individual level, and harder when all the data are grouped. Person-specific information is important as a source of material for reflection. This includes feedback about communication skills and patient empowerment, including the empathy, respect and facilitation of coping strategies by the doctor.

Other questions are more related to service delivery, whose results tend to lie more outside the appraisee's sphere of influence. Over time, all appraisees should be encouraged to seek individual data.

Paperwork facilitation skills

Facilitation has been defined broadly in terms of appraisal as 'helping appraisees think through where they are now, what they want and need in order to develop as professionals, and how to organise themselves to achieve it', as described in Chapter 3.

All the other skills described here contribute to the new appraiser's ability to do this. For the purposes of the training curriculum, it has been defined more narrowly as the skills required to facilitate the production of a comprehensive, accurate and useful Form 4 and a well-designed, achievable and motivational PDP.

Writing a good Form 4

It is important that appraiser training highlights the vital nature of Form 4 as one of the outcomes of appraisal. Appraisers will wish to have a clear understanding of what should and should not be included. Some guidance on writing a good Form 4 is covered in Chapter 8.

Appraisers may wish to debate who should write the Form 4 in order to ensure that it is factually correct and owned by the appraisee as their record of their appraisal. The government guidance says that it should be written by the appraiser and agreed by the appraisee, but in some areas whoever can type fastest or write most legibly completes the form.[22] Elsewhere, local policies clearly state that it is the appraisee's responsibility to fill it in.

There may also be a debate on whether the Form 4 and the PDP should be completed at the time or whether it is acceptable to take them away to complete after reflection. It is desirable to complete them while both signatories are together at the time of the appraisal, as a further level of negotiation on content can then take place. In circumstances where this has proved impossible, it is imperative that the completion and sharing for signature are done as quickly as possible so that the momentum is not lost.

Facilitating a good personal development plan

The other key outcome of appraisal is the PDP for the coming year. New appraisers need a good understanding of how to facilitate a useful and effective PDP as described in Chapter 8.

This is an area where practising with good and bad examples and using tools for the assessment of the PDP can be very useful in training. The new appraiser will rapidly gain a feel for what is unacceptable, acceptable and excellent. The PDP produced in any given appraisal will be dependent to some extent on the appraisee. An experienced appraiser will not be dispirited by this but will have the skills to help produce something that is meaningful to the appraisee.

Dealing with difficult appraisals

There are some common scenarios that cause concern for all appraisers. Having the chance to rehearse them through role play in appraiser training, and later on in ongoing support group sessions, builds confidence. It allows the appraisers to demonstrate their competencies in the communication skills required to break down barriers and establish rapport.

Appropriate scenarios can easily be written to target training on specific skills. Some of the situations that create anxiety are listed in Table 5.4.

Common appraisee pitfalls

The appraiser's skills can be severely tested when the appraisees' behaviours seem to stem from innate attitudes that are a hindrance to their achievements and aspirations. The paperwork for appraisal can also challenge the appraiser in various ways. Too much or too little paperwork may make preparing adequately difficult. On the other hand, the paperwork produced for just one year seen in isolation may not be an accurate reflection of the documentation the appraisee has produced over time. It can occasionally be useful to ask whether previous appraisal documentation can be seen if there appear to be concerns or adverse trends. Sharing the previous paperwork may be particularly useful when there is a change of appraisers.

Table 5.4 Types of appraisee

Preparation	Attitude	Special cases

• Too much paperwork
  – organised
  – disorganised
• No paperwork
  – good Forms 1–3
  – poor Forms 1–3
	• The high flyer
	• The overcommitted
	• The unbeliever
	• The cynic
	• The imminent leaver
	• The insecure
	• The dependent/
	  disempowered
		• The poor performer
		• The ill
		• The whistle blower

Below are some examples of these issues, with suggested questions that might be suitable to provoke self-reflection.

Table 5.5 Too much paperwork: organised

Characteristics	Challenges
• Reminds you of your most obsessional patients • The paperwork requires an elephant to transport it • Two weeks hardly seems like enough to read it through • Hard to see the wood for the trees • Leaves appraiser feeling inadequate about their own documentation/depressed	• How did you decide how much evidence to submit? • How do you prioritise your work? • How would you assess this supporting documentation? • What do you think is the most important piece of work/evidence/documentation in here . . . why? • Help me to home in on what really interests you . . .

Table 5.6 Too much paperwork: disorganised

Characteristics	Challenges
• Reminds you of your most disorganised colleague • The paperwork still requires an elephant to transport it • Two weeks hardly seems like enough to read it through • Seems to want you to do all the work of sorting it out • Extremely hard to see the wood for the trees • Some paperwork can be very unrelated to the appraisee	• How did you decide which paperwork to give me? • Do you feel that more structure to your supporting documents would be useful? • How can we prioritise what we need to discuss? • What is the most important document here? . . . and the least?

Table 5.7 No supporting evidence: good Forms 1–3

Characteristics	Challenges
• Forms 1–3 excellent, but no supporting documentation • It all sounds wonderful and probably is but there are no specific examples available to discuss • Appraiser feels unable to prepare adequately	• I am very impressed by the time and effort you have put into Forms 1–3. What sort of documents do you think you could have used to back up the statements in Form 3? • It is hard to discuss this without a specific example. Could you suggest one? • Do you keep your supporting documentation elsewhere? May I see it? • What documentation would you have liked to include? • I feel I have not been able to prepare adequately because there was so little supporting documentation . . .

Table 5.8 No supporting evidence: poor Forms 1–3

Characteristics	*Challenges*
• Forms 1–3 poor, and no supporting documentation • It all seems very flimsy and insubstantial • Leaves the appraiser feeling anxious about this appraisee • Appraiser feels unable to prepare adequately	• It appears to me that you have not spent much time on your preparation. Is there a problem? • It is hard for me to help you without more to discuss. Are there any burning issues for you? • What documentation would you have liked to include? • I feel I have not been able to prepare adequately because there was so little supporting documentation . . .

Table 5.9 The high flyer

Characteristics	*Challenges*
• Has a long list of achievements and successes • Often has local, regional or national influence • Demonstrates a great deal of achievement drive • May not have a great deal of reflection on weaknesses • Leaves the appraiser feeling insecure about their own ability	• Looking at all these impressive achievements, which means the most to you, and why? • Do you still feel driven to achieve more? Why? • Are you aware of the ways in which you use your influence? • Is there anything you would like to do but you feel you could never succeed at? • How do you feel about revealing your weaknesses? • Where do patients come in your order of priorities? • I feel rather inadequate when I look at all you do. How do you think the other members of your department/practice feel? • Within and beyond your professional activities, do you feel that anything important is being sacrificed on the altar of your success? • How do you feel about your work/life balance?

Table 5.10 The overcommitted

Characteristics	*Challenges*
• Between all the different roles (including family) there don't seem to be enough hours in the week • May be frequent comments about lack of time in the paperwork • May be evidence of failing to deliver or complete on things • Seems stressed • Makes the appraiser feel tired	• You do so much. Do you feel you manage to fit it all in OK? • What has to give in your life for you to deal with this workload? • Have you ever felt you couldn't deliver on a commitment you had made? How did that make you feel? Can you think of anything you could have done differently? • With all these commitments, it must be quite stressful . . . (pause)

Table 5.11 The unbeliever

Characteristics	Challenges
• Criticises the appraisal process • Criticises your experience to appraise him • Criticises everything to your face (but writes a glowing evaluation afterwards and says he would like you again) • Leaves appraiser feeling anxious that nothing useful was achieved	• You seem very negative about the appraisal process. What upsets you about it? • I feel that you were rather I were not your appraiser . . .? • I am feeling that I am not able to do a good job here. Is there anything I could change to make it more useful for you? • What have we achieved that feels worthwhile?

Table 5.12 The cynic

Characteristics	Challenges
• Views appraisal as a hoop to be jumped through but with no power to affect things • Can sometimes be persuaded otherwise by the power of the experience itself • Can become strong advocate of the process afterwards • Leaves the appraiser feeling (a) powerless if still unconvinced or (b) fantastic	• You seem to feel appraisal is merely a hoop to be jumped through . . . (pause) • I'm sorry you feel like that. Do you know of anyone who has found it a positive experience? • Let us try together to make this time as useful as possible for you. What are your top priorities this year?

Table 5.13 The imminent leaver

Characteristics	Challenges
• Very dismissive of the whole process • Has not spent any time preparing their own paperwork • Says clearly that appraisal is an irrelevance to them • Has significant overlap with the cynic	• You seem to feel appraisal has no relevance to you . . . (pause) • I'm sorry you feel like that. Do you know of anyone who has found it a positive experience? • Let us try together to make this time as useful as possible for you. What are your top priorities this year? • There are ways to use your appraisal to strengthen your departure planning . . . (pause)

Table 5.14 The insecure

Characteristics	Challenges
• Doesn't recognise their own strengths • Focuses on weaknesses at all times • Has rarely if ever had this much personal attention focused on their work and very threatened by it • Needs a great deal of encouragement • Often insecure about running to time • May have been hurt by a complaint in the past • Leaves the appraiser feeling very tired (but usually happy)	• What do you feel was your greatest achievement this year? • What impressed me in preparing for this appraisal was . . . • What type of case do you feel you deal with best? • You keep coming back to areas you find difficult but I want you to focus first on what you do well . . . • You seem insecure about your abilities but in my experience this is supporting documentation of a very high standard . . .

Table 5.15 The dependent/disempowered

Characteristics	Challenges
• Seems very helpless when faced with paperwork • Keeps looking to the appraiser for answers • Finds it hard to make decisions • May seem disempowered within the clinical environment too • May be being bullied by a colleague • Makes the appraiser feel either (a) irritated or (b) useful and needed • Appraiser feels that they are doing all the talking (reversing the intended 80/20 split)	• How do you feel you could take control of this appraisal? • I feel you are looking to me for answers. What are your priorities? • How do you make decisions? Not just at work but in your life outside work too? • I have the feeling you have felt unable to take control here . . . • What do you feel about bullying? Have you ever had any experience of it? • When you ask me what I think you should do, it makes me feel a bit irritated because I feel this is your appraisal and I shouldn't be giving you the answers . . . • I feel that I am being very useful to you, but what do you feel that you should be contributing here? • I wonder whether I am doing too much of the talking here . . .?

Table 5.16 The poor performer

Characteristics	Challenges
• Extremely rare • Finds that in the freedom of the appraisal a deeply held anxiety can find expression • Blurts out (usually) something that has not even been hinted at in the paperwork • May get very emotional • Makes the appraiser feel concerned for the appraisee and for patient care	• What you have just said is really serious. Let's take a bit of time outside the appraisal to explore that . . . • You seem very upset. Do you need a break? Would this be a good time for me to go and get us both a drink? • This seems to be outside the bounds of the appraisal discussion. Shall we stop the appraisal here for now? • You know that what you have just said has implications for patient care . . . (pause) • I am glad you have felt safe to reveal that. I am here to support you in working through what to do next . . . (pause) • You know I will have to report this discussion because it affects patient care. We need to put things in place for you to be able to stop now . . . • What do you think we should do next?

Table 5.17 The ill

Characteristics	Challenges
• Very rare • May present in a similar way to a poor performance issue • Finds that in the freedom of the appraisal a deeply held anxiety can find expression • Blurts out (usually) something that has not even been hinted at in the paperwork • May get very emotional • Makes the appraiser feel worried about the appraisee and sometimes about patient care	• Any of the challenges used for the revelation of poor performance, plus . . . • You have obviously been worrying about this for some time . . . (pause) • You seem to be telling me that you are seriously ill . . . (pause) • Who else knows about this? Do you feel able to tell your colleagues/partners/spouse/a friend/your GP? • What would you be telling someone else in your position to do?

Table 5.18 The whistle blower

Characteristics	Challenges
• Brings a serious concern about a third party to the appraisal discussion • May seem to want the appraiser to 'do something' or to 'pass the buck' to the appraiser • May know what needs doing and just want the chance to talk it through • Can leave the appraiser feeling (a) irritated at being given unwelcome information or (b) able to empower the appraisee to deal with it	• This is a very serious accusation about your colleague. What are the implications? • May I ask why you have raised this? What were your expectations? • What do you feel your responsibility should be here? • What you have told me is hearsay, but do you have evidence that needs acting on? • Do you know about the whistle-blowing policy locally?

Summary

In practice, appraisees do not conform to stereotypes (unless they are choosing to play a single role). Difficult appraisals will usually involve a mixture of some of these attitudes. The high-flying appraisee may also produce too much meticulously organised paperwork and then reveal that it is all fuelled by alcohol as a stress reliever.

Being an appraiser is a privilege, but it is not easy and there are no perfect answers. It is important that training relieves anxiety sufficiently to allow new appraisers to feel well prepared for the role, while allowing them the freedom to experiment and find their own style. This process parallels the method by which inexperienced doctors become trained in consulting skills, which they apply initially by rote (conscious competence). Through experiential learning and feedback, particularly by looking to learn from real or simulated consultations, the conscious use of skills can develop into unconscious competence with the increased flexibility this provides. The use of real and simulated appraisals is an equally powerful tool for appraiser training.

Training new appraisers: attitudes

Self-awareness

Consideration of the need to be self-aware has led to the recognition of some personality traits and prior skills that might lay the appraiser open to particular temptations or traps. These are encapsulated in the statements below.

Common appraiser pitfalls to be aware of

The 'nice guy'

As an appraiser, I have to be especially aware that I like to be liked and find it hard to be controversial or give negative feedback. I am very good at being supportive but I feel I am sometimes not challenging enough.

The elder statesman

As an appraiser, I have to be especially aware that I have had a very senior role for many years and I find it hard to avoid giving the appraisee the benefit of my considerable experience. It can be difficult to give them enough time to find the answers for themselves even though I know that it will mean more to them if they do.

The teacher

As an appraiser, I have to be especially aware that I have had so much experience as a teacher or trainer in a one-to-one setting that I sometimes slip back into the teacher role rather than facilitating the appraisee's own reflection. Some appraisees ask me to tell them the answer and it is tempting to do so when I feel that I know it. The appraisal lead has commented that my PDPs are recognisable as my appraisees often include learning tools that I am keen on.

The diffident

As an appraiser, I have to be especially aware that I feel very inexperienced compared with some of my senior colleagues when I am required to appraise them. I worry that they won't take me seriously and therefore won't get the most out of their appraisals. I also find it hard to challenge individuals who are influential in my local area. I have felt threatened or bullied by an appraisee.

The task oriented

As an appraiser, I have to be especially aware that I am very good at focusing on the task of getting through the appraisal on time and with all the correct paperwork completed accurately. I risk sometimes missing out on the more subtle clues an appraisee gives me that they have something else to discuss.

The colluder

As an appraiser, I have to be especially aware that I believe that causing problems for my colleagues will make the recruitment and retention problems even worse and so I am tempted to try to make appraisal as easy and painless as possible. For example, I like a drink or two, so it is hard to challenge people if they raise the amount they drink in the health section.

The critical

As an appraiser, I have to be especially aware that I can see the holes in the evidence provided all too clearly and find it hard to raise the awareness of the appraisee in a way that does not seem too harsh or 'holier than thou'. I dislike leaving a gap even when the PDP includes quite enough for one year.

> **The doctor**
>
> As an appraiser, I have to be especially aware that I am not doing my day job and trying to solve individual's problems for them by eliciting the relevant history and then making recommendations. I can be tempted to use tools for assessing depression or drinking that really belong in my clinical practice. I know that the appraisee knows them too, so I have to be careful not to move from appraisal to consultation mode.

> **The over-involved**
>
> As an appraiser, I have to be especially aware that I can find it difficult to maintain my detachment. I have been known to stray into a counselling role and have even offered follow-up sessions with me when I know I should have signposted other forms of help.

Being self-aware

Acknowledging that these personal stumbling blocks exist is the first step towards ensuring that they do not get in the way of delivering an effective appraisal. Rehearsing alternative strategies within an appraisal support group and discussing difficult appraisals after they have occurred (again in terms of process, not specific content) can lead to useful insights.

Freedom from bias and prejudice

In the real world, none of us can be entirely free of bias and prejudice. Our cultural background gives us terms of reference that we are often largely unaware of. The purpose of training is to bring our everyday assumptions into the arena within which we are self-aware so that we can deal with them appropriately. If an appraiser normally works on the assumption that all doctors are altruists, who do their jobs because they have a vocation, then that is a bias that will be carried into appraisals. It may make it harder for him to deal with a doctor who is very cynical or works only for the money.

Becoming aware of our personal prejudice can be a painful process and needs to be handled carefully in the training.

Non-judgemental

Being non-judgemental is an essential attitude for creating an environment where an appraisee feels comfortable. Appraisers are not there as policemen or judges and it should never feel as if they are.

Constructively challenging

The appraiser needs some guidance in appraiser training about the level of challenge that is appropriate and how best to be constructive. Appraisees do not like to spend their time on a process that is insufficiently challenging:

> I wanted to be able to really explore my ideas with my appraiser, not have a 'yes man' agreeing with all my proposals.

All challenge can be threatening, as a need to change is implied. Constructive challenge is specific, respects the appraisee, moves the agenda forwards and highlights behaviour that does not seem congruent. Appraisers reflect what the appraisee has articulated (which may well differ from what is in the hidden agenda) and what they have observed. By bringing conscious and subconscious fears and thoughts into the open, it allows them to be explored and addressed.

An equally important skill is that of returning to territory that is comfortable and secure for the appraisee before moving on to other areas and new challenges. This is often called 'getting back to safe ground', and can be achieved through speaking about things that are now agreed and not contentious.

Supportive and understanding

If the ethos of appraisal as a supportive developmental process is ingrained in the appraiser training, then being supportive and understanding should follow naturally into facilitating real appraisals.

Situations will arise where the ability to be supportive is hard. Sometimes appraisers appraise more than one person in the same team and know that there is more than one side to a story. In the appraisal of one individual, however, that appraisee needs to be heard and supported to develop.

It may be tempting to try to get to the 'truth'. Who would this help? Truth is a very elusive thing as it depends so much on perception. The appraisee can be challenged to consider the situation from a different point of view and encouraged to reflect on how to develop skills to manage issues better, but this will only work in a supportive, not a judgemental or critical, environment.

Professional

From an appraiser's point of view, professionalism must be about taking personal responsibility for becoming and remaining as skilled as possible. Each appraisal should be performed as though it was being assessed, drawing on all that the appraiser can offer. Each appraisee is important to their own patients and deserves a positive and useful appraisal with real outcomes in terms of professional development.

Sometimes, appraisers can blame themselves if they feel they have not been able to conduct an appraisal to such exacting standards. Professionalism is also about realising that not every appraisal can go perfectly. It takes both parties to make an effective appraisal.

How the curriculum should be evaluated

Appraiser training providers need to have an assessment process that is transparent and fair. Potential new appraisers should have person specifications to measure themselves against, and a clear understanding of the contents of the medical appraiser curriculum. At the outset of training, it should be explicit that they will not be recommended for appointment if they fail to meet minimum standards of competency in all the key areas. Role play, example paperwork, contributions to the discussions and attitudes demonstrated during training can all play a part in informing the decision about suitability for the role. The feedback from the first supported appraisal has been a particularly valuable assessment tool in some training courses.

Whatever the assessment methodology is, candidates must have the opportunity to demonstrate their competence to the best of their ability. If a candidate is not recommended for appointment, it is good practice for the training providers to provide a detailed debrief about the competencies that have not been demonstrated.

Just as different training providers will have particular preferences about how to teach individual skills, so each programme should be designed with specific outcome measures in mind. The aims and objectives of each course should be specified in advance and the means of assessment made clear to participants.

Because appraiser training was so variable in the early stages, there may be great variation in the quality and standards of existing appraisers. There needs to be a robust quality assurance process for ongoing skills updates. This will allow those who are unable to demonstrate the required skills to be performance managed and prevented from continuing in a role for which they do not have the right knowledge, skills or attitudes. The evidence that a bad appraisal is damaging and dangerous (and worse than no appraisal at all) is clear.[23]

Conclusion

A curriculum for appraiser training has been discussed in terms of key knowledge, skills and attitudes. Appraisal training providers will want to ensure that all the core areas are adequately covered and that every new appraiser feels confident to undertake the first supported appraisals. The assessment of whether an individual has succeeded in demonstrating the key competencies will allow the training providers to make a recommendation on appointment to the employing organisation. Only those candidates who have successfully demonstrated appropriate levels of knowledge, skills and attitude should be able to become appraisers.

Once appointed, appraisers should be required to demonstrate that they are maintaining and developing their competence in all the key areas. This might be done through annual skills update training and assessment sessions, combined with direct feedback from the appraisals done during the year. Those who cannot meet the required standards should not be allowed to continue appraising.

References

1   NHS Education Scotland. *GP Appraisal Scheme: a brief guide*. Edinburgh: NHS Scotland; 2003.
2   Chambers R, Tavabie A, Mohanna K, Wakley G. *The Good Appraisal Toolkit for Primary Care*. Oxford: Radcliffe Medical Press; 2004.
3   National Clinical Governance Support Team. *Assuring the Quality of Training of Medical Appraisers*. Leicester: NCGST; 2006.
4   Spady W. *Outcome-based Education: critical issues and answers*. Arlington, VA: American Association of School Administrators; 1994.
5   General Medical Council. *Good Medical Practice*. 3rd ed. London: GMC; 2001.
6   Royal College of General Practitioners. *Good Medical Practice for General Practitioners*. London: RCGP; 2002.
7   NHS Appraisal Toolkit. *Appraisal Toolkit Guidance*; 2003. www.appraisals.nhs.uk (accessed 19 August 2006).
8   Jacques D. *Learning in Groups*. 3rd ed. London: Kogan Page; 2000.
9   National Clinical Assessment Service. *Roles and Responsibilities in Addressing Concerns About the Performance of GPs in England Agreed by COGPED and NCAS*. London: NCAS; 2005.
10 GP Appraisal and CPD Unit. *GP Appraisal in Wales: annual report 2004/2005*. Cardiff: Cardiff University School of Postgraduate Medical and Dental Education; 2005.
11 Burns R. To a mouse. Unknown.
12 Rughani A. *The GP's Guide to Personal Development Plans*. 2nd ed. Oxford: Radcliffe Medical Press; 2001.
13 Middleton P, Field S. *The GP Trainer's Handbook*. Oxford: Radcliffe Medical Press; 2001.
14 Eve R. *PUNs and DENs: discovering learning needs in general practice*. Oxford: Radcliffe Medical Press; 2003.
15 Attwood M, Curtis A, Pitts J, While R. *Professional Development: a guide for primary care*. Oxford: Blackwell Publishing; 2005.
16 Howard J. *An Evaluation of the Higher Professional Education Scheme for General Practice in Mersey Deanery*. Liverpool: Mersey Deanery; 2003.
17 Royal College of Physicians. *Doctors in Society: medical professionalism in a changing world*. London: RCP; 2005.
18 Schon D. *The Reflective Practitioner: how professionals think in action*. 2nd ed. Aldershot: Arena; 1991.
19 McMorran J, Crowther D, McMorran S, Prince C, YoungMin S, Pleat J. *GP Notebook*; 2006. www.gpnotebook.co.uk (accessed 19 August 2006).
20 Greco M, Carter M, Powell R, Sweeney K, Stead J. Does a patient survey make a difference? *Educ Prim Care*. 2004; **15**: 183–9.
21 National Primary Care Research and Development Centre. *General Practice Assessment Questionnaire*. Manchester: NPCRDC; 2003.
22 Essex Appraisal Steering Group. *GP Appraisal in Essex: the Essex scheme*. Chelmsford: Essex Appraisal Steering Group; 2002.
23 Murphy K, Cleveland J. *Understanding Performance Appraisal*. London: Sage; 1995.

Chapter 6

Preparation for appraisal

This chapter deals with the responsibilities of the appraiser in preparing for the appraisal discussion. It describes Forms 1–3, and how to look at the supporting documentation. There is guidance on some practical details of preparation.

> Failure to prepare is preparing to fail.
> **Unknown**

Introduction

The preparation for an individual appraisal begins as soon as an appraiser and an appraisee are paired. The tone of the whole appraisal discussion is set, in part, by the success, or otherwise, of the process that leads up to it. To avoid negative first impressions, because they lessen the potential for a really effective appraisal, the organisational set up must be smooth and efficient.

Appraisees need to feel respected and valued and sense that the appraisal is given priority by the organisation. There is, therefore, a real need for adequate administrative support from a team that is fully committed to formative, developmental appraisal. The organisational culture will have a significant impact on the way that appraisees value their appraisals.[1]

Getting the process going

Most appraisees will begin to think about their appraisal when the appraisal discussion is booked. There may be a structure for the appraisal process in place that the appraisee and appraiser are meant to follow. Unfortunately, appraisees vary widely in their knowledge of, and adherence to, such systems and the appraiser and administrator cannot assume that they know what will happen from the booking onwards. Those who are newly appointed will particularly appreciate a reminder.

It may be very helpful to share a timetable for the appraisal process at the time of setting up the appraisal. Local systems can vary substantially but it is good practice to clarify who has responsibility for particular aspects of the local administration.

In some models, it may be the responsibility of the secretary or administrator to set up a suitable time and venue for the appraisal, with the appraiser and appraisee both being notified separately. Other models have the appraiser and appraisee liaising directly to co-ordinate what can be very complicated diaries.

It is prudent for the final arrangements, however they are agreed, to be put in writing and sent electronically. When there are last-minute changes, it is even more important that everyone, including the organiser or administrator, and both the appraiser and appraisee, are kept informed.

Box 6.1 The contents of the appraisal confirmatory letter

A confirmatory letter should include:

- the date, time and location of the appraisal
- a reminder about privacy, freedom from interruptions and the amount of time to set aside
- the responsibility chart
- arrangements for the sharing of the forms and supporting documentation
- details of the system for keeping documentation secure
- the appraiser and appraisee contact details

plus:

- the procedure for using the NHS Appraisal Toolkit,[2] if used
- a cancellation clause.

Details to be confirmed

Any confirmation should highlight the date, time and venue for the appraisal discussion (Box 6.1). It should also make explicit the amount of time that needs to be protected and the need for privacy. It will be necessary to include contact details for both the appraiser and appraisee, plus any stated preferences about the easiest way to make contact. The details about how to safeguard the appraisal documents are very important. Both appraiser and appraisee must share the same understanding of how and where documents will be delivered in order to make sure that confidential paperwork is protected.

A confirmation letter could also include a reminder of the procedure for signing off the NHS Appraisal Toolkit[2] and to bring passwords and log-on details to the appraisal, if the Toolkit has been used.

Cancellation clause

There needs to be a standard reminder of the consequences of a late cancellation of the appraisal. For portfolio clinicians, agreeing to do an appraisal at a particular time may preclude them from taking on other fee-earning work. Other doctors may have employed a locum to free their time. Under what circumstances this money will be reimbursed, and by whom, should be clear at the outset.

Timetable for the appraisal process

Throughout the year
- Continuing professional development (an ongoing and cyclical process).

Two months before
- Agree date and venue.

One month before
- Finalise paperwork.

Two weeks before
- Documentation securely received by appraiser.
- Electronic paperwork signed off online by appraisee.

Before the appraisal
- Preparatory work by appraiser.

On the day
- The appraisal discussion.

After the appraisal discussion is complete
- Complete paperwork.
- Secure storage of public documents.
- Collation of responses and evaluations.

At the end of the year
- Production of annual report.

Throughout the year
- Continuing professional development.

Where to meet

The location chosen for the appraisal itself is highly variable. Almost anywhere that meets certain basic requirements may be appropriate. These requirements are summarised in Box 6.2.

Box 6.2 Requirements for a suitable venue for appraisal
- Acceptable to both parties
- Comfortable
- Quiet
- Free from interruptions
- With necessary equipment: online access, computer, printer, photocopier
- Essential facilities

It is paramount that the location and timing of the appraisal are acceptable and convenient for both parties. Arrangements that are perceived as unfair will make it difficult for both individuals to arrive on time and in a relaxed frame of mind. Privacy is essential to creating the environment of confidentiality that will allow free discussion of potentially sensitive issues. This need obviously precludes an appraisal from being done in an open-plan office or, as in the apocryphal stories, in the pub.

The location must be quiet and allow both parties to feel comfortable. A stifling small room on a hot day in the summer cannot be recommended. It is important that there are appropriate facilities available. In particular, appraisees who have chosen to use the NHS Toolkit for Appraisal[2] will be frustrated if there are no facilities to go online and create the summary of the appraisal discussion and the personal development plan at the end of the discussion. Even those not using a Web-based system may need access to a computer and a printer, as well as a photocopier. This equipment needs to be considered when choosing a venue. It may go without saying, but, as the appraisal is likely to take a significant length of time and effort, adequate facilities for natural breaks and refreshments should also be considered.

Many clinical directors and GPs will choose to host the appraisal in their own offices or consulting rooms. This can be very helpful if it means that supplementary documentation and appropriate facilities are to hand. However, it is important that the person who is not on their home territory is able to feel equally relaxed. It is also vital that there is a guarantee of freedom from interruptions. For this reason, some GPs, in particular, make a point of requesting a location away from their own practice.

If the normal office or consulting room is chosen, then a sign should be put on the door to remind those who might otherwise forget, not to interrupt. It is a good idea for both parties to switch off their mobile phones, as they can be guaranteed to ring at the most intense and inappropriate moments.

Sometimes the location is a neutral venue organised by the appraisal administrator or secretary. Successful appraisals have even been held in the appraiser or appraisee's own home, but only if a suitable room is available, the other requirements can be met and the choice is acceptable to both parties.

When to meet

The main priority for the timing of the appraisal is that it is mutually convenient for both the appraiser and appraisee. Neither should feel anxious about something else that is going on elsewhere, or aggrieved, or it will be impossible to create the atmosphere of respect and trust required. If there is a personal crisis going on, it may well be appropriate to acknowledge this and put it consciously to one side as part of the preliminary housekeeping.

It is essential to allow adequate time for the appraisal process. It is particularly unfair if the appraisee feels they have not been given the time they expect and deserve.

It is also strongly recommended that no fixed commitments are scheduled immediately after the appraisal. If done well, it is likely to have created food for thought. It requires time to process and reflect on these ideas before stepping back onto the treadmill of everyday life. Both the appraiser and the appraisee should allow this flexibility at the end, as the discussion can have an equal impact on both (Box 6.3).

Box 6.3 Requirements for the timing of an appraisal

- Mutually acceptable
- Adequate time for housekeeping
- Adequate time for the appraisal
- Adequate reflection and processing time afterwards

Producing Forms 1–3 and the supporting documentation: how long should it take?

Continuing professional development (CPD) is an ongoing process that should not have a maximum time put on it within the bounds of achieving a satisfying and fulfilling work–life balance. At different times in their career and different life stages, doctors will inevitably have more or less time and energy to spend on CPD. The doctor doing a Masters may put in huge numbers of hours for a couple of years and then reduce dramatically when the first child comes along.

Although the appraiser does not have a policing role, it may be useful to consider during the preparation of the paperwork how much CPD activity appears to have been undertaken. Feeding back to a very driven appraisee that 50 hours of CPD is the recommendation from many of the Royal Colleges, and that they seem to be doing much more than necessary to keep up to date, may liberate them from the constant anxiety that they are not doing enough.

It is fair that part-time clinicians should have to do an equal amount rather than proportionally less than their full-time counterparts. Arguably, because they are getting less experiential learning it is even more important for them to keep up to date.

From the point of view of helping an appraisee to prepare for revalidation it is also vital to challenge those who appear to be doing very little. Sometimes this is because a wealth of learning activity that is perfectly legitimate has not been considered as such and is not included. Sometimes life events have intervened. Such appraisees need support from their appraiser to be able to demonstrate at least 50 hours of activity in subsequent years. If individual work and private study can be counted, rather than solely attendance at specific accredited educational events, then this total does not seem unreasonable.

The initial guidance in primary care was that the completion of the paperwork should take a session of clinical time (3.5 hours).[3] Many doctors found that it took significantly longer because they were unused to collecting information suitable for appraisal. However, as time goes on and doctors become familiar with the process, the annual appraisal documentation itself becomes less of a chore. Much of the material can be collected in one place over the course of the year, and the reflection becomes more embedded in day-to-day work, rather than being a single task at the year-end. This can be done electronically with the NHS Toolkit or other software, or by having a dedicated paper file for the supporting documents as they are produced.

Appraisers should be supporting the appraisees in what they choose to bring to appraisal and in ensuring that they are aware of the need to record 50 hours of CPD. Asking how long it has taken to pull all the paperwork together can give useful insights to both parties.

Safe dispatch of paperwork

The paperwork and supporting documents put together by the appraisee can be very private and informative. Each appraiser/appraisee pair needs to agree how they will share the pre-appraisal documentation to ensure its security. It may be handed over personally, delivered by recorded delivery or retrieved from a safe haven within the trust. The detail is unimportant, as long as both parties are satisfied that the confidentiality of the paperwork has been safeguarded.

How to look at the forms and paperwork

Once the appointment for the appraisal discussion has been booked, and the appraiser receives the documentation from the appraisee, the major part of the preparatory work for the appraiser starts.

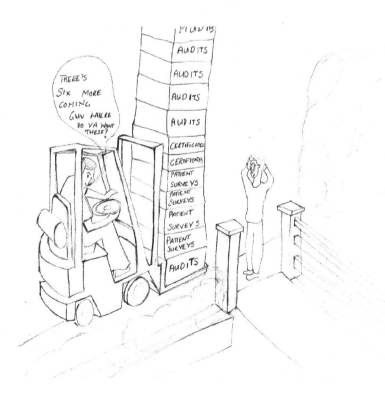

While reading the documentation it is important for appraisers to attempt as far as possible to clear their heads of any bias or prejudice they may have. This applies whether the perceptions are positive or negative.

It is rare for an appraiser to know nothing at all about the person they are appraising. This prior knowledge needs to be brought into the conscious awareness in order to be dealt with appropriately. An appraiser who believes that a colleague is part of a dysfunctional team within the hospital may bring unhelpful preconceptions to the appraisal. Denying that the prior knowledge exists is even more likely to be detrimental than acknowledging it and bringing it into the open.

Preparing stem questions and themes

The appraiser may find it very useful to have thought through some key open questions that will lead the discussion along. If the flow of the appraisal is going well, then these may not be needed, but if it stalls then the effort put in prior to the appraisal itself will certainly pay off. Helpful types of questioning are covered in detail in Chapter 7.

Examples of open stem questions to tackle the problems of preconceptions:

- 'I have heard that your team is having a few problems at the moment. How do you see the situation?'
- 'Because I have heard some gossip, I was wondering how you would describe relationships within your team at the moment?'

Or an open statement:

- 'I was interested to see what you put about working with colleagues because I had heard that your team wasn't working so well at the moment . . .'

These could be perceived as very challenging and give rise to:

- 'Who told you that? What makes them think so?'

Or to a more open response:

- 'Yes, we would get on so much better if communication links could be worked out.'

Even the defensive response can lead to another avenue to explore:

- 'You seem very defensive about your team . . .' (pause).

A key lesson is not to enter the trap of responding to the defensiveness.

Preparing the documentation

Many appraisers start their personal preparation by doing a preliminary read-through from beginning to end of Forms 1 to 3 without necessarily exploring any of the supporting documentation. This gives an overview of the appraisee's ideas and helps to place the appraisee's clinical work and professional development in context.

With this in mind, the appraiser can then start the detailed preparation. Often the previous year's Form 4 and PDP are a good starting point. If they have not been included, the appraisee should be contacted before the appraisal to be reminded, as signing off the PDP is essential as part of the appraisal. This gives the appraisee who has forgotten to include them a chance to retrieve them and allow the appraiser to have a copy in advance. If the previous documentation is not available, the appraiser and appraisee will need to be prepared to discuss this during the appraisal.

A walk through Forms 1–3 of the standard paperwork is included below. Within these, the appraiser will be looking out for areas that might be highlighted for discussion. In particular, the appraiser will be looking for:

- a point to open the session and start relationship building
- areas where something innovative or excellent practice has been described
- areas where the appraiser has not recorded any activity or the information is incomplete.

Form 1: basic details

Form 1 includes all the biographical details about the doctor. It lays out name, address and contact details, qualifications and details of GMC registration, and asks about the date of the last revalidation. It looks at the date of appointment to the current post, a description of that post and any other posts held currently or within the past five years. It also asks for other relevant personal details, including membership of professional bodies. It should be brief and factual and will only need altering from year to year if there is a material change.

It can be tempting to skim over Form 1. Particularly where the appraiser has prior knowledge of the appraisee, there can be an assumption that all that is here is already known. In practice, there are often interesting openings for the discussion as individuals may have qualifications the appraiser did not know of, or be a member of a society that reveals something new. The description of the current and previous posts (within the past five years) can also be a rich source of information.

Form 2: current medical activities

Form 2 is the place to record an overview of the types of work that an individual undertakes. Form 2 for GPs starts by asking about the number of hours per week worked. In both primary and secondary care, the form asks for in-hours and emergency, on-call and out-of-hours work to be described separately. It has a space for details of any other clinical work and any other NHS or non-NHS work that is non-clinical but undertaken in the capacity of doctor. It asks about work for regional, national and international bodies, and any other professional activity. Despite the title of the form, most appraisees do include all their non-medical activities here too.

This form should also be brief and factual and will only vary a little from year to year as individuals take on new responsibilities or change the range of activities they undertake. It gives the appraiser an essential insight into the shape of the appraisee's working life, although there is little in Form 2 to identify which of all the things they do are important to the appraisee.

Not preparing Form 2 thoroughly can lead the appraiser into deep water in the appraisal. Appraisees assume that the appraiser will know what they do from what they have put here. In fact, there is rarely enough detail because of the way the form is constructed. Clarifying some points at the beginning of the appraisal can be a useful opener. It shows the appraisee how much has been prepared and allows the appraiser to more fully understand the range of activities undertaken.

Form 3: material for appraisal

As appraisees, all doctors need to consider their strengths and weaknesses, how they have already developed and what development needs they have for the future. They also need to look at the constraints upon their ability to practice and a way of feeding back information about all these things to their employing organisation. The layout of each heading under 'Form 3: material for appraisal' encourages exactly this reflection. The government forms also include some useful hints on what might be included in each section.

Discussion of the reflections recorded here and the supporting documentation provided by the appraisee form the largest part of the appraisal discussion. Without any evidence of reflection or adequate supporting documentation, the appraiser has very little to prepare. At the outset of appraisal this was not uncommon. Part of the appraiser's role was to help the appraisee identify how to approach appraisal in order to get the most out of it and what to collect. Wise appraisees want to ensure that their appraisal folder contains all the evidence they are likely to need for revalidation in order to avoid duplicating effort and to assure themselves that they are performing as well as they believe.

Now that almost all appraisees are familiar with the process and have been supported by their first appraisers in considering how to make the documentation as useful as possible, the quality of the reflection and supporting evidence should be improving. If it were not, reflecting on that might well be a very important area for the appraiser to tackle with the appraisee.

Critical reading skills include the ability to:

- identify significant inclusions
  - examples of excellence
  - examples of problems
- identify significant omissions
- read between the lines.

Good clinical care

Good clinical care is the section in which appraisees aim to demonstrate their clinical ability as doctors. Reflection on the main strengths and weaknesses of clinical care is the cornerstone of the appraisal. Discussing what has improved since the last appraisal and what constraints there are on the appraisee are less emotive than discussing what does not go so well. Yet appraisees want to be challenged effectively and are grateful to have the chance to reflect on areas they find difficult.

> If my appraiser hadn't challenged my ideas, the appraisal discussion would all have been a waste of time as I wouldn't have moved forwards from what I had worked out for myself in my preparation.

In preparing the good clinical care section, the appraiser will be looking at the supporting documentation provided under this heading as well as what the appraisee has written. Are the statements of strengths backed up by evidence or are they assertions with no demonstrable verification? Has the appraisee included a statement about complaints during the year or any details of a complaint? Are there significant event analysis or critical incident reports? Has there been any sort of audit that has evidence of personal involvement by the appraisee, or reflection on the results?

The appraiser must be looking for examples of excellence as well as significant omissions. Asking for more details about an example of good practice may lead to a suggestion that the idea be shared more widely, for example, in a best practice forum. When something does not appear to be present, making a note to ask about it is not the same as creating a required list of evidence (which the English system does not yet have). It can be a useful prompt to the discussion.

> For example, 'I notice you haven't said anything about complaints. Does that mean you had none during the year? Don't you think that that is significant negative information that you would like to record?'

Maintaining good medical practice

This section looks at the appraisees' systems for keeping up to date and abreast of their professional development. Most appraisees seem to find this the easiest section to record and include all sorts of certificates and evidence of attendance at events. Fewer include reading diaries or learning logs and fewer still have kept reflective notes.

Appraisees should be encouraged to summarise their professional reading and record membership of any action learning sets or small groups they are involved with (e.g. a journal club, a young principals group). Last year's Form 4 and PDP may well be included here.

All appraisees should be:

- reflecting on their practice (though they may not be conscious of doing so)
- undertaking some opportunistic learning
- undertaking some structured learning.

Many appraisees are unaware of how many different educational opportunities they use. Historically, they would not label much of what they are doing as learning. For example, in chatting with colleagues over coffee about a troublesome case, a doctor can be changing their understanding of how best to manage the patient. It can be an important function of the appraiser to reflect back to the appraisee the learning that the appraiser has become aware of, both during preparation and during the appraisal discussion.

Another area to prepare is how to engage appraisees in reflective practice in a way that would be meaningful and useful to them. Some consideration of useful tools is given in Chapter 5.

Merely listing educational events attended has long been discredited in educational circles as providing any evidence of actual learning taking place. 'Bums on seats' do not necessarily correlate with 'minds actively engaged'. Appraisees should always be encouraged to record at least one point of reflection on anything they attend or do in order to learn. Even if it says 'This course was boring and had no new information', a useful discussion about how to choose better which courses to attend may result.

Relationships with patients

Being required to reflect on relationships with patients is an important area of professional life. Most doctors believe that they have good relationships with their patients. It can be very challenging to try to demonstrate that that belief has substance. It is also hard to demonstrate that relationships have improved year on year, or to identify further areas for improvement if the feedback is already very good. Being encouraged to reflect on it at least once a year is a very positive discipline.

Some doctors may be used to videoing their patient interactions, or working with actors, to improve their consultation and communication skills. Reflection on this sort of activity can be very fertile ground for discussion. Other doctors will include patient survey data, from tools such as those described in Chapter 5 or appreciative letters and cards.

This type of feedback provides useful openings for the appraisal. If there is no documentation to back up the assertions the appraisee has made, part of the appraiser's role is to facilitate the recognition that such evidence would be useful, and how to collect it.

Relationships with colleagues

Being required to reflect on relationships with colleagues is as important as looking at relationships with patients. Doctors are often aware of tensions in their working relationships, which they do not address. They may feel it is more effort than it is worth, or they may feel disempowered to change anything. A chance to reflect, in confidence, can reveal that a problem is not as big as previously thought and can put an appraisee's anxieties to rest, or it can empower the appraisee to take action that would have seemed to difficult without the opportunity to talk it through.

It can feel even harder for an appraiser to prepare the section on relationships with colleagues than the section on relationships with patients because the guidelines on supporting documentation are even less clear. There may be good evidence of team meetings and the sharing of audit data, or participation in a supportive group. A few appraisees will have asked for feedback specifically on a particular area of practice, e.g. their referrals, or on their role within the team, sometimes using 360-degree or multi-source feedback tools (as described in

Chapter 5). Practice in looking at the outcomes of such tools will help the appraiser prepare effectively.

A lack of supporting documents will give the appraiser an opening to discuss how impressions about relationships with colleagues are arrived at, and how to gather appropriate feedback. It seems likely that such documentation will be one of the areas considered for revalidation,[4] so any process that helps in its collection will be useful.

Teaching and training

Most doctors, from medical school days, are aware of the old adage 'See one, do one, teach one'. Things have moved on and now there are skills laboratories and very realistic models on which to practise clinical skills. Actors and simulated patients offer opportunities to rehearse communication skills in particular. Many doctors are involved in some form of teaching and training from the formal clinical lecturers, to the informal registrar supporting his senior house officers. While doctors in training themselves form a subgroup of extraordinary appraisees, this section is likely to have some resonance for almost all.

Any appraisee who takes part in teaching and training activity should include a summary of what exactly they do. These factual data need to be understood by the appraiser. The next area for discussion is reflection on the teaching or training activities, which might include evaluations from learners or peer review of a teaching session. By preparing carefully, even those appraisers who are not teachers or trainers can usually facilitate these reflections successfully.

Management

It is useful to consider management activity separately from clinical care because the knowledge, skills and attitudes needed to be successful can be significantly different. The development needs in this area may be very important for the smooth running of the organisation or team.

Appraisees use this section to describe any formal (usually remunerated or backfilled) management activity they undertake. A clinical director has significant management responsibilities. Primary care organisations have specific clinical leadership roles, e.g. GP Professional Executive Committee (PEC) member.

Appraisees do not usually describe their management activity within their own practices as GPs, or their own clinical team, indeed the form suggests that only management outside should be included. However, sometimes significant management skills are needed within the appraisee's core role too, and a discussion can be useful.

Research

Not all doctors carry out any research to record in this area. It is not uncommon for there to be a comment about 'no formal research activity' and no plans to do any. The perceived difficulty of getting ethics committee approval for projects means that many doctors shy away from the idea of research.

However, it can also be an area of concern for appraisers when the appraisee does do research, if the appraiser feels ill-equipped to facilitate the reflection. Awareness of concern may lead to a suggestion that there be a joint appraisal to cover this area of the appraisee's work, or another expert be asked to contribute on a separate occasion to the appraisal. There may be a local organisational research team lead, whose details could be included in the appraiser's pack under useful contacts.

A few appraisees undertake significant amounts of formal research and may need a special appraisal model (*see* Chapter 9). Some are happy for the clinical appraisers to cover this section too, in which case the appraisers may review the papers and reports that inform the supporting documentation. Unless it is relevant to them, they may not read every word of a research article that has been peer reviewed and published. What the appraiser does need is the overview of the research interests of the appraisee to facilitate the discussion and to help the appraisee ensure that research complies with ethical guidelines.

Health

There has been significant uncertainty on the purpose and usefulness of the health and probity sections of the appraisal paperwork. Some recent work has suggested that appraisers see it as a 'wasted opportunity'.[5]

'Are you in good health?' 'Yes!' is clearly not a meaningful exploration of this potentially rewarding area for discussion. In some ways, the health and probity sections seem to be included because they are main headings in *Good Medical Practice*[6] and to be useful primarily in preparation for revalidation. Confusion has arisen because there is no route by which appraisers can act as policemen in these areas, and nor would they want to. In the appraisal discussion the appraiser takes at face value what the appraisee chooses to present.

Evidence for good health cannot therefore come from the appraisal process. This evidence could be in the form of a suitable self-declaration.[1] The only other options would be true health assessments by the appraisee's own GP or an occupational health physician. Both of these would have major resource implications for the health service and undermine the principles of professionalism. The only significant piece of evidence that is now being provided routinely in some areas is the hepatitis immunisation record. Keeping it in the appraisal documentation and reviewing it each year is a useful way for many doctors to ensure it is kept up to date.

Because it can be seen as threatening to consider health issues, the facilitation provided by a trained supportive appraiser in confidence can be a unique opportunity for an appraisee to acknowledge a concern. Flagging up risk factors and providing signposts to appropriate resources can hopefully help to prevent health problems. Even where a health problem exists, appraisal may provide a unique opportunity to talk through the implications and make safeguards for patient care.

Reflection on how appraisees look after their ongoing health, both mental and physical, is often facilitated by careful preparation. The appraiser might prepare a quick checklist based on the requirements of *Good Medical Practice* under this heading and explore each briefly with the appraisee. Significant omissions, like hepatitis B immunisation status, should be highlighted for mention during the appraisal discussion.

If the appraisee feels there are no health-related issues that might put patients at risk, or that the issues have been adequately explored, they will usually feel able to include a suitable signed self-declaration about their health.

If there has been thorough preparation, carried through into the appraisal discussion, by the end of the appraisal, the appraiser will be able to sign off this section of the paperwork with confidence, knowing that the issues have been thought through and appropriate precautions put in place. Many doctors have chronic health problems and an annual consideration of the implications for their work is an appropriate safeguard for patients.

Probity

Although some of the concerns around the probity section echo those for health, particularly about it being impossible to police and probably being more related to revalidation than appraisal, it is an even more emotive issue for many doctors. Appraisal would not have identified Dr Harold Shipman, because he was a clever criminal but not an incompetent doctor, and it is not designed to seek out criminality. This point has often been made, most emphatically by Dame Janet Smith.[7]

Moving beyond concerns about revalidation, some of the advantages to having an opportunity to discuss areas of uncertainty or concern about probity issues in confidence during the appraisal should be re-emphasised. Most doctors are confused about the definition of probity. Prior to the advent of appraisal, it is unlikely that many had read *Good Medical Practice*.[6]

If the appraisee feels there are no probity-related issues that might put patients at risk they will usually include a signed self-declaration about their probity. The appraiser might prepare a quick checklist based on the requirements of *Good Medical Practice*[6] under this heading and explore each briefly with the appraisee.

The safeguards that are in place to ensure propriety in financial and commercial affairs might include declaration of interest forms, statement of criminal convictions, Criminal Records Bureau (CRB) checks, etc. Significant omissions are worth reflecting to the appraisee who may not have been aware of the value of collecting such data and keeping it in the appraisal folder.

The overviews

This final section of Form 3 has three parts:

- overview of development during the year
- overview of development needs
- overview of constraints.

It can be one of the most fruitful areas to prepare. If the appraisee has considered these areas carefully then a large part of the appraisal and the subsequent PDP will already be defined. The appraiser should be prepared to challenge what has been put in here if it does not seem to be a full reflection of the development needs apparent from the rest of the paperwork. There may also be a need to reflect back to the appraisee those things that have not been included.

Being seen to be prepared

It is not merely important to be prepared, it is helpful if it is apparent to the appraisee during the appraisal discussion that the appraiser has read and thought about the documentation. This is often revealed by the specifics that the appraiser recalls and uses as examples during the discussion. Unless appraisers have photographic memories, however, they will also find it useful to make notes.

Some areas have devised standard preparation forms, which give a structure for taking notes and recording the supporting documentation, an example of which can be found in Chapter 11. Creating notes made during the preparation, during the discussion and on reflection all on the same sheet leads neatly to having the right information to hand to write or type up the Form 4 under the headings of *Good Medical Practice*.[6]

Others may have inserted markers into the paperwork with comments relevant to that section or have another system of their own devising. The exact structure does not matter. It is important that the appraisee is aware of the preparation that the appraiser has done and feels that their preliminary work has been adequately considered and valued.

Notes during the discussion

As part of the chair function, the appraiser should take notes during the appraisal to act as an aide memoire and ensure that no significant strands of the discussion are lost. Individuals differ in their ability to take effective notes while concentrating on facilitating the appraisee's reflections. Nevertheless, a few bullet points make all the difference at the end to ensuring that the Form 4 can be accurately completed.

Notes during reflective time

Some appraisers find it very helpful to have a break in the appraisal between the discussion phase and the completion of the paperwork. During this time for reflection, they may make further notes to address with the appraisee at the time of writing up the Form 4 and PDP.

Potential issues relating to the documentation

What if the forms are not backed up by appropriate supporting documentation?

Historically, a lot of the content of Forms 1 to 3 consisted of assertions by the appraisee, which were not backed up by supporting documentation. For example, many appraisees might state that they were 'good listeners' as a clinical strength, without any evidence to back up this self-assessment.

Is this an issue? The initial appraiser training made it absolutely clear, in England at least, that the content of the appraisal discussion should be owned by the appraisee. It is a process designed to allow them to explore issues fully and frankly, and it was anticipated that they would not feel enabled to do that if they also felt the appraiser had a policing role. Many appraisers have felt inhibited from asking for supporting documentation in case they were seen as judgemental.

In practice, this is a false assumption. Appraisees want accurate feedback in order to benchmark themselves against their peers. On the whole, they welcome the challenge of being asked how they know that an assertion is true. Often there is evidence available but they have not realised that it could or should be included with the appraisal documents. Sometimes the challenge leads to a decision to produce the evidence as part of the next year's PDP.

Most appraisees are now aware that there will be a requirement to produce some kind of portfolio of evidence for revalidation. Why produce two separate portfolios when the support of the appraiser can be invaluable in creating a file of valid and useful supporting documentation that serves both purposes?

Whose appraisal is it anyway?

It is quite clearly the appraisee's appraisal and the appraiser's job is to facilitate their self-reflection. But it is also the organisation's appraisal, because one of the outcomes is an amalgamated list of learning needs identified and constraints on practice which is presented to the trust board. Getting the documentation right is key to helping the information gained to be accurate and specific enough to be actionable. Recommendations arising from appraisal need to be acted upon if the process is to deliver value for money and important outcomes like improvements in patient care.

What information is necessary?

The minimum information that the appraisee must provide is fully completed Forms 1 to 3. If these are not completed, the appraiser can reasonably conclude that the appraisee is not engaging in or committed to the process of appraisal. As appraisal is a statutory requirement, this conclusion has serious performance implications.

There are a few situations that give rise to special considerations in responsible organisations. These include maternity leave and prolonged sick leave. Without such a mitigating excuse clinicians could find themselves in some form of disciplinary procedures for not engaging in annual appraisal.

What information is desirable?

The types of supporting documentation that can be used to back up the statements made in Form 3 in particular are discussed elsewhere. Currently, nothing is essential and, equally, nothing included by the appraisee is likely to be useless unless it relates to a team effort in which the appraisee had no personal involvement. Even then it may be fruitful to explore why the doctor chose to include it.

How can the information be supplemented?

For most appraisals, the appraiser works solely with the portfolio presented by the appraisee and does not seek to find out more. However, if the appraisee seems to have sent unusually little supporting documentation, it may be worth making contact and making them aware of this before the appraisal date. It is surprising how often more could have been sent or is brought to the appraisal when there is no time to prepare it properly. A quick phone call or email can often prevent this and allow the appraiser time to work with the supporting documents.

Occasionally, the organisation within which an appraisee works produces a portfolio of useful evidence and makes it available to the appraiser. For example, some areas produce practice profiles for GP practices, detailing information about demography, achievements and difficulties, which are also made available to appraisers. In secondary care, some clinical directors have a huge amount of performance management data available to them about the practice of the clinicians within the directorate. Such information needs to be shared with the appraisee before the appraisal documentation is prepared so that reflection upon it can be included in Forms 1–3.

What if a third party presents privileged information and expects it to be acted upon during the appraisal?

Suppose that a clinical governance lead has come to an appraiser and described an outstanding complaint against a doctor and asked the appraiser to address it during the appraisal. This scenario has led to significant anxiety and discussion in appraiser groups. Once known, the information cannot be unknown again. The appraiser therefore will tackle the appraisal in a slightly different frame of mind and certainly with a different understanding of the environment in which the appraisee works. The response to such a request has been divided into distinct strands.

Organisational

- A clarification for the benefit of the clinical governance lead of the confidential and appraisee-led nature of the appraisal discussion.
- A clear refusal by the appraiser to agree to manipulate the agenda of the appraisal.
- A similar clear refusal to feed back to the clinical governance lead anything that transpires during the discussion that is not included on the agreed Form 4 and PDP.

Personal

- An acknowledgment that this information is now in the open and an awareness that it will lead to a hypersensitivity to areas that may lead to discussing the complaint in question.
- An acknowledgment that the appraisee may be desperate to have the chance to talk the issues through in the protected environment of appraisal but needs to be reassured of the level of confidentiality first.
- An acknowledgement that, just as some patients start by denying that they have cancer and refusing to discuss it, an appraisee might be in the denial stage and not yet be able to process issues relating to the complaint.
- An acceptance that it is OK to discuss it (despite the fact that the initial awareness came externally) and equally OK not to discuss it and that the choice must rest with the appraisee.

Before the appraisal appraisers should share with the appraisee what they have been told, and their response about the formative and confidential nature of appraisal. This would put the control back with the appraisee to choose whether or not to continue to discuss the complaint, knowing that it would be confidential and would not be fed back to the clinical governance lead.

It is best practice for the appraiser also to let the clinical governance lead know what they are planning to share with the appraisee.

Last-minute changes/additions by the appraisee

Having shared the documentation with the appraiser two weeks earlier, the appraisee may have thought of something else that they wish to bring to the appraisal. It would seem inappropriate not to allow an individual the right to do this, but an appraiser would also be within their rights to ask for time to consider any new submissions before starting the appraisal proper, or even to postpone the appraisal if it appeared the appraisee had presented a substantially new portfolio that would require a lot of preparatory time to do it justice.

The last-minute checklist: the appraiser

Before setting off for an appraisal, the appraiser will wish to conduct a mental review of the things they need to take and consider (Box 6.4). The appraisal is the opportunity to return all the documentation that the appraiser has received, including Forms 1–3, with all the initial reflection and any supporting evidence from the appraisee. It is also important to remember the preparatory notes that the appraiser has made, as any such notes must afterwards be considered the property of the appraisee and returned to them for shredding or to keep (depending on how useful they find them).

Sometimes electronic copies of the blank paperwork, on a CD ROM or memory stick, etc., might be useful.

A note of necessary log-ins and passwords if they are not memorable will be important if the online resources are to be used effectively.

Box 6.4 Pre-appraisal checklist for the appraiser

- Appraisee's documentation
- Preparatory work
- Appraiser's pack
- CD ROM/memory stick
- Appraiser's log-on details and passwords for the online Toolkit, etc.
- Directions to the venue
- Contact details for the appraisee

The appraiser pack

In many areas there will be a local appraiser pack, which should be taken to every appraisal. Suggested contents are listed in Box 6.5.

Box 6.5 The appraiser's pack contents

- Blank paperwork, including:
  - official forms
  - evaluation forms
- Useful telephone numbers and websites
- Contact details for local educational resources
- Appraisal policy document, including:
  - details of whistle-blowing procedure
  - procedures for dealing with doctors in difficulty
  - occupational health scheme
- CD with electronic copy of all the appropriate paperwork and resources

---

Punctuality

Appraisals can be derailed entirely by one or the other party arriving late and creating an atmosphere of haste and tension. The appraiser should remember to print off the directions to the venue if it is unfamiliar. It may also be useful to carry a contact number for the appraisee, just in case. Being in next-door offices in a trust building and unable to find each other would be very frustrating.

My appraisal was delayed for a whole hour because of a last-minute venue change, so I went to a different place from my appraiser.

Conclusion

Preparing thoroughly for an appraisal is vital. The organisation and structure of the appraisal meeting will set the tone for the discussion that takes place. The work that the appraiser has done beforehand will contribute to making the appraisee feel valued. Critically reading the supporting documentation is an essential skill in facilitating the development of the appraisee and it improves with practice. When an appraiser arrives at the appraisal discussion relaxed and confident of being well prepared, the stage is set for the most effective appraisal possible.

> You cannot prepare enough for anything.
> **James Galway**

References

1   National Clinical Governance Support Team. *Assuring the Quality of Medical Appraisal: report of the NHS Clinical Governance Support Team Expert Group.* Leicester: National Clinical Governance Support Team; 2005.
2   NHS Appraisal Toolkit. *Appraisal Toolkit Guidance;* 2003. www.appraisals.nhs.uk (accessed 19 August 2006).

3 Department of Health. *NHS Appraisal: guidance on appraisal for general practitioners working in the NHS*. London: DoH; 2002.

4 Chief Medical Officer. *Good Doctors, Safer Patients*. London: DoH; 2006.

5 Whittet S. Health and probity in appraisal: what do you ask? 2005 [accessed 30 April 2006]. Available from: www.appraisalsupport.nhs.uk

6 General Medical Council. *Good Medical Practice*. 3rd ed. London: GMC; 2001.

7 Lyons N, Leigh P. Shipman 5: the implications for medical educators. *Educ Prim Care*. 2005; 16: 111–14.

Chapter 7

The appraisal discussion

This chapter explores the appraisal discussion, and how to make it a success. It is crucial the central part of the appraisal is effective. An adaptation to the Calgary–Cambridge consultation model is presented as a way of considering how the appraiser may wish to lead and facilitate the process.

> The unexamined career is not worth having.
> (Misquoting Socrates 470–399 BC 'The unexamined life is not worth living')

Introduction

The face-to-face interaction between the appraiser and appraisee has been deliberately called 'the appraisal discussion' as opposed to 'the appraisal interview'. This is to underline the fact that it is a not a hierarchical interaction during which summative assessments are made. It is a dialogue during which appraisers facilitate appraisees to reflect on their work, their strengths, their weaknesses and the constraints that may affect them as doctors (who are also human beings).

In Chapter 6, the appraiser was taken through the skills and tasks needed to prepare for the appraisal. The most auspicious ingredients for a successful discussion, after preparation, are punctuality and time keeping. Arriving in good time gives appraisers time to collect their thoughts and acquire a flavour of the appraisee's place of work. Observing how the appraiser is welcomed and how the members of staff interact with each other and the appraisee is interesting. It may well make the appraiser aware of issues not raised in the appraisee's paperwork (The 'blind spot' of the Yosuni appraisal windows described in Chapter 2).

This also gives appraisers the final chance to decide whether they have sufficient information to embark on the appraisal. There may have been initial agreement that all, or some, of the supporting evidence would be presented immediately prior to the appraisal. If the appraisers feel that there is not sufficient information on which to base an effective appraisal discussion, they need to decide how to handle this and whether to attempt to proceed or not.

> I know that we have worked in the same patch for over 10 years and I am aware of your achievements and standing. However, do think it will do you justice . . . I mean, will you have a really professional appraisal if we continue today without your folder of evidence . . .?

Chapter 5 explores this and other difficult appraisal situations that may arise.

Calgary–Cambridge model

The framework advocated for any appraisal discussion is an adaptation of the Calgary–Cambridge guide to the medical interview (Figures 7.1 and 7.2).[1] Its advantages include the fact that an appraisal discussion has many similarities to a consultation with a patient. Appraisers will already have in their consultation toolbox a chart and a raft of skills, which will need minimal editing for the appraisal process.

It is essential to remember that the structure described in this chapter is only a suggestion to help the appraiser. The process has to be appraisee led.

For less-experienced appraisers, and appraisees in particular, a proposed structure for the proceedings can be supportive and confidence building. If weather and road conditions are good, the traveller may not need to refer to a map at all. If there is an unexpected diversion, visibility becomes poor or the vehicle develops mechanical problems, a map with useful phone numbers and local information suddenly becomes vital.

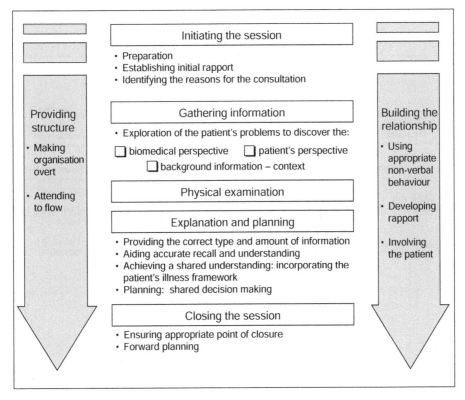

Figure 7.1 The Calgary–Cambridge guide: the expanded framework (for the medical interview). Reproduced with kind permission from Kurtz *et al. Teaching and Learning Communication Skills in Medicine.* Oxford: Radcliffe Publishing; 2005. © Kurtz *et al.*

The essential stages for holding a useful appraisal discussion, based on the Calgary–Cambridge guide, are:

- initiating the session
- providing structure
- building the relationship
- exploring the appraisee's statements, ideas and aspirations
- agreeing the Form 4 and PDP
- closing the session.

Certain communication skills are vital for all stages of the appraisal discussion. They are particularly useful when exploring the appraisee's statements, ideas and aspirations. They will be discussed after a brief consideration of these six steps.

Initiating the session

The well-prepared appraiser will find initiating the session a reasonably smooth process. The first step is to establish initial rapport. If the appraisee does not know

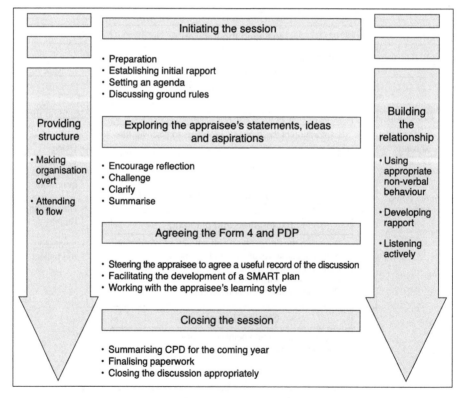

Figure 7.2 A guide to the appraisal discussion based on the enhanced Calgary–Cambridge guide to the medical interview. Adapted by Dr A McEwen with kind permission from Kurtz *et al. Teaching and Learning Communication Skills in Medicine.* Oxford: Radcliffe Publishing; 2005.

the appraiser it is important to make proper introductions. An initial chat, bringing in some of the information the appraisee has given, begins relationship building and creates a relaxed, trusting atmosphere.

A successful meeting needs an agenda, skilled chairmanship and an outcome of clear action points.[2,3] The agenda will have been partly set by the paperwork and supporting documentation. It is reasonable for the appraiser to have drafted some points to explore with the appraisee before the meeting. This has been addressed in more detail in Chapter 6. It needs to be emphasised that the draft agenda must support an appraisee-led process rather than impose the appraiser's ideas on the proceedings.

In order to use time efficiently, it is good practice to refine the agenda before the discussion gets underway. It is helpful to find out if there is anything the appraisee wishes to discuss that may have arisen since the documentation was completed. There may be issues that the appraisee felt were too sensitive to record prior to the appraisal. This strategy, as in the consultation, helps to avoid the discussion being prolonged or reopened when it appears that it is coming to a conclusion. It can pre-empt the so-called 'door handle' comment: 'By the way . . .'.

> Effective use of time is achieved by checking as far as possible at the beginning of the discussion that there is no new important material that the appraisee wishes to introduce, and that the most significant issues are discussed in a timely way.

It is vital to consider the seating arrangements for the discussion wherever possible and with agreement of the appraisee. Positioning the appraiser and appraisee in a

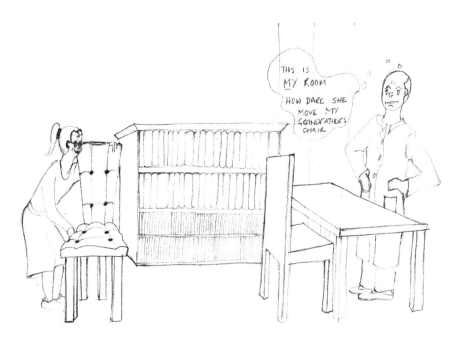

way that is comfortable for both parties, facilitates note taking and does not create any hierarchy is useful in setting the atmosphere of the appraisal discussion. There is good evidence from medical consultations that careful consideration of the seating arrangement can affect the outcome.[4] It seems reasonable to assume that the same applies to the appraisal discussion.[5]

Providing structure

Providing structure and building the relationship need to be woven throughout the appraisal discussion. They can be viewed as the pillars on which the other skills rest and the backdrop against which the discussion takes place. They are discussed here as part of initiating the session, as they must be present from the outset.

The initial pleasantries serve to give the appraiser an idea of the appraisee's commitment to the appraisal process. This helps the appraiser to judge what sort of approach to take, how to pitch the discussion or, indeed, whether to start the appraisal at all.

Thankfully, most appraisals start without a hitch, and once the initial small talk is over, the appraiser needs to signal the beginning of the formal process. Negotiating the structure of the session helps the appraisee to know what shape the discussion might take. To make this explicit, the appraiser needs to establish whether the appraisee is comfortable with the order in which the appraiser proposes to discuss things.

- Introductions.
- Negotiating the probable length of the appraisal discussion.
- Turning mobile phones off and establishing the possibility of any unavoidable interruptions.
- Agreeing if and when a break might be taken.
- Are there the facilities and the will to use the NHS Appraisal Toolkit?[6]
- Clarifying the confidentiality rules and who will have access to the Form 4.
- Reminding the appraisee of the procedure should previously undiscovered poor performance issues arise.
- Negotiating the way in which notes will be taken to inform the final documentation.
- Deciding who will do the typing/writing. (The guidance[7,8] says the appraiser will fill in the Form 4, but common sense dictates that the fastest typist or more legible writer should be the scribe, as long as what is written accurately reflects what has been discussed and agreed.)
- Discussing this year's preparatory work (Forms 1–3 and last year's PDP) and the need to sign them off.

While structure is necessary for planning the appraisal discussion, to ensure important issues and necessary tasks are addressed, it should not control the process so that it detracts from the flow of the discussion. Flexibility is the key, particularly if the appraisee becomes distressed or emotional.

Building the relationship

In discussing the above topics, the appraiser will have demonstrated some skills to the appraisee. In turn, the appraisee will have made some decisions about the appraiser and formed a view of how things might go.

The appraiser needs to invest effort in building a special relationship of trust and mutual respect. This allows the giving of negative feedback and challenge to the appraisee appropriately. There might be a prior relationship between the appraiser and appraisee. This needs to be acknowledged and the appraiser needs to behave in a way that sets the professional tone of the discussion. The appraiser needs to pay regular attention to the developing relationship, diffusing any tensions that arise and trying to ensure the atmosphere is one in which the appraisee can think, share and reflect.

If the discussion is initiated well, the appraisee may be able to explore more sensitive issues in depth. If the appraiser has been insensitive and done something without mutual agreement, the tone of the whole appraisal may have been destroyed, and there may be difficulty in rebuilding the relationship.

Initiating the session well, therefore, is a crucial first step in smoothing the progress into the next phase of the discussion. It is worth spending time and effort on providing structure and building relationships at this phase.

In another model of the consultation, Roger Neighbour[9] combines the ideas of 'building the relationship' and 'initiating the session' as 'connecting'. Building on a good connection between the appraisee and appraiser will make the appraisal discussion easier and more productive.

Exploring the appraisee's statements, ideas and aspirations

In exploring the documentation that the appraisee has provided, the appraiser has the privilege of taking the appraisee on a voyage of self-discovery. There are essential tasks to be undertaken. More significantly, a set of skills are needed in the appraiser's toolbox to facilitate a journey that challenges well-established thinking and behaviour, while reaching the agreed destination in good time. While these tasks and skills overlap, they will be discussed separately below to assist understanding.

Agreeing the Form 4 and PDP

Whoever types or writes the Form 4 and PDP, it is crucially important that the appraisee owns everything in the document. This may require negotiation, and may be done throughout the discussion, rather than at the end. In this way, the important valuable outcomes of the appraisal are not rushed. Sometimes it may be necessary to defer finishing the paperwork if the appraisee needs more time to reflect and consider things.

> ... I knew I wouldn't get that [an action on his PDP] done, but my appraiser insisted that I put it in and as we were running out of time, I agreed.

Appraisers should remember that the Form 4 is an important document that needs to be filled in with care.

If the total time and effort spent on the appraisal is to be cost-effective and useful, the Form 4 must be an accurate, legible and meaningful summary of what transpired during the appraisal discussion. It should help appraisees in their reflection. Throughout the next year, they will need to keep a record of their achievements and aspirations alongside a clear picture of their goals.

In negotiating what goes into the Form 4, the appraiser has a duty to ensure that it is an accurate distillate of the discussion. It should give a flavour of that discussion as well as recording the factual content. Some appraisers list the supporting evidence that has been presented. The PDP is discussed in Chapter 8.

As with the Form 4, the appraiser needs to agree with the appraisee a PDP that really does RUMBA[10]:

Relevant
Understandable
Measured
Behaviour change
Achievable.

The Form 4 and PDP are sent to the responsible person (clinical governance or appraisal lead) in the NHS organisation to which the appraisee is accountable. Organisations vary as to whether these forms are sent to the next appraiser. These forms are like a 'baton' being handed on from one year to the next. This allows continuity and helps to inform the appraisal discussion. Appraisers and appraisees can then, to some degree, look at the past, the present and the future.

Closing the session

If all the paperwork has been completed, this section of the appraisal may be quite short. It should be clarified who is responsible for getting the forms to the designated person in the organisation. Depending on the system prevailing in the area, a six-month contact may or may not be agreed.

The appraiser needs to make it explicit that the role does not include retaining any paperwork about the appraisee. It is also good practice to remind the appraisee of the need to keep the documentation for the future.

Despite the best of intentions, some appraisal discussions simply overrun the allotted time. Some appraisees are deeply reflective and prefer to contemplate the PDP before finally agreeing it. The information technology (if, for example, the Form 4 and PDP are being recorded electronically) may fail halfway through, or delay may occur for other unavoidable reasons. If the paperwork is deferred for any reason, it is worth discussing exactly how and when the Form 4 and PDP will be agreed and signed off. Clear timescales need to be negotiated. The appraiser should not feel that the job is done until the whole process, including the paperwork, has been wrapped up neatly.

Evaluation forms (examples in Chapter 12) should be used. These provide the appraisers with valuable information about their performance.

It is important that the appraiser encourages the appraisee to complete the evaluation forms. It is helpful if the appraisee knows why the forms need to be filled in, who will receive them and how the results will be fed back to the appraiser. There should be an option for anonymity. In some areas, the appraiser also fills in an evaluation of the appraisal. This is compared with the appraisee's view of the appraisal as a way of enriching the feedback to the appraiser.

Finally, it is only polite to thank the appraisee for their time and hospitality.

Signing off the previous year's PDP

Looking at last year's PDP should be used as an opportunity to help appraisees recognise their successes and focus on their priorities. It is worth acknowledging what appraisees have achieved in the preceding year. This should not be a box-ticking exercise but a genuine acknowledgement of accomplishment. In the face of constant change in the way doctors are expected to work and demonstrate their competencies,[7] achieving the goals individuals set themselves can be a major triumph. After all, 'appraisee' does contain the word 'praise'.

Encouraging the appraisee to reflect on the PDP planned in the previous year against what has actually been done, and why, is a powerful but temperate way to 'dig deeper' and stretch the appraisee. If a target has not been met, then the reasons are worth exploring.

The appraiser could choose to challenge (dealt with later in this chapter) or decide it is too early in relationship building and just listen and defer comment until later.

Together, the appraiser and appraisee need to decide what is still relevant and needs carrying forward and what may be dropped in the light of the appraisee's current needs. It is also useful to explore whether any achievements need further development. Health professionals tend to undertake education in topics they are already good at or interested in, rather than in what their learning needs dictate.[11]

Discussion of Forms 1, 2, 3 and 'any other business'

The skills that might be employed to facilitate the discussion of these forms and, importantly, any other areas the appraisee may choose to bring up, are the most important part of the appraiser's toolbox. They are addressed below.

Skills for facilitating the appraisal discussion

Having considered the stages involved in the appraisal in terms of the adapted Calgary–Cambridge appraisal guide, it is now important to discuss the communications skills that are especially relevant to facilitating the appraisal discussion.

1 Non-verbal communication
   – paraverbal communication
   – body language
   – picking up cues
   – mirroring.
2 Questioning
   – Socratic
   – open
   – closed.
3 Reflecting.
4 Challenging.
5 Getting back to safe ground.
6 Demonstrating empathy.
7 Signposting.
8 Encouraging reflection.
9 Active listening.
10 Summarising.
11 Giving feedback.

I Non-verbal communication

Mehrabian[12] found that about 7% of the impact of a message is verbal, while 38% is paraverbal (vocal) and the remaining 55% is non-verbal. Birdwhistell[13] similarly estimated that the verbal component of a face-to-face conversation is less than 35%, leaving over 65% to be done non-verbally.

We now consider some aspects of non-verbal communication that an appraiser should learn to read and interpret in order to maximise the effectiveness of the appraisal discussion. The appraiser needs to decide whether to act on the non-verbal message immediately or wait for a more appropriate moment.

Paraverbal communication

Paraverbal communication can be described as the signals with which words are dressed. They include:

• pauses
• tone of voice
• volume
• speed
• emphasis on different words.

In the appraisal discussion, as with many communication situations, pauses are very useful. A pause allows both parties to gather their thoughts and formulate what they are going to say. This enhances the effectiveness of the communication. A pause by the appraiser can replace a question. A pause from the appraisee may denote many things: uncertainty; a desire not to develop a particular line of discussion; or a need to stop and just be. A pause should not be prolonged for the sake of it but, in reality, they are usually shorter than they appear to be.

The tone of voice, volume and rate of speech, and the emphasis placed on particular words are all important aspects of paraverbal communication.

If an appraisee increases the volume of speech, the appraiser should reflect on the possible reasons for this and resist the natural inclination to mirror the appraisee and also increase the volume.

Body language

There are many elements of non-verbal communication and a few pertinent ones are considered here.

Eye contact is important, but the appraiser needs to be aware of personal variations and cultural norms in relation to this. In some cultures, it is unacceptable for a woman to look anyone other than a close relative in the eye. Behaviour change is always difficult and non-verbal communication is no exception. There is, therefore, the potential for doctors from other cultures to find their hard work in learning the language diluted because it takes even longer to adjust to the indigenous way of non-verbal communication. This will affect the appraisal as much as it does the doctor–patient interaction. Similarly, a shy or unconfident individual may communicate less in every way, including non-verbally. Not every appraisee who avoids eye contact is depressed or lying.

Gestures are an important aspect of non-verbal communication and need to be interpreted in context. Many are culturally or genetically determined,[14] some being universally understandable such as shrugging shoulders to denote ignorance. Other gestures can have different meanings in different parts of the world. For example in some cultures the word 'yes' or the non-verbal message 'I am listening to you' is signalled by shaking the head from side to side, while in the UK that would mean disagreement.

Picking up cues

Cues may be verbal or non-verbal and both types are dealt with here as they accompany each other both in the giving and the receiving of messages. It is usually important to check verbally with the appraisee that the appraiser has read the cue (verbal or non-verbal) correctly.

> **Appraisee:** 'Don't get me wrong, I enjoy everything I do, but (pauses) I do wonder . . .' (tails off).
> **Appraiser** (after a suitable pause): 'I get a sense that you have some conflict about your workload at the moment, is that something you wish to discuss?'

The reader can imagine the body language that might accompany the appraisee's statement above.

The skill of picking up cues would be in noticing the hesitation, the appraisee perhaps looking away or shifting position and the voice tailing off, which could denote uncertainty. It is important to read silences carefully; the appraisee may be a deliberate speaker who simply needs time to choose his words.

As the majority of communication is non-verbal, it should be remembered that non-verbal communication may need to be given more weight than the actual words used when a discrepancy is apparent.

Mirroring

At the outset of the appraisal discussion, the appraiser and appraisee may not have closely shared goals. During agenda setting, it is important that the appraisee receives the message that the appraiser is 'on side' and wants to be 'with' rather than 'against' the appraisee.

Mirroring is feeding back what the other is telling you using non-verbal language. The purpose of mirroring is to let the appraisee know that the appraiser is willing to really listen and understand the appraisee's point of view.

Matching or parroting[9] are other terms used for mirroring, and this is done by subtly matching the appraisee's non-verbal language; their body movements, posture, gestures, tone of voice, etc. This is usually done subconsciously and can be observed in any situation where people are having a positive interaction. It is important when practising this skill that the appraiser does not mirror in an exaggerated manner. This would be distracting for the appraisee and might cross the line into mimicry, which is unacceptable.

2 Questioning

Apart from appropriate non-verbal behaviour to encourage open and honest discussion, the appraiser's questioning technique is all important.[10]

Usually three kinds of questions are described:

- Socratic
- open
- closed.

The above classification provides a useful way of discussing the use of questions in the appraisal discussion, but the boundaries are not rigid and the appraiser needs masterly questioning skills in order to ask the right question at the right time in the right way.[15]

It is worth reflecting on the paradox posed by Mackay[16] that the minute that the question has been asked, the questioner becomes the listener.

Never miss a chance to shut up . . .
Will Rogers (1879–1935)

Socratic questions

These questions follow the method of Socrates, asking incremental questions to facilitate the other person to find answers for themselves. During Socratic questioning, the questioner demonstrates a model of critical thinking while respecting the other person's viewpoints. Socratic questions probe understanding, and show genuine interest in the other person's thinking. The questioner creates and sustains an intellectually stimulating environment and acknowledges the value of the appraisee in that environment. In an open, safe and demanding appraisal, appraisees will be challenged, yet comfortable in answering questions honestly and fully.

Open questions

Open questions do not allow a 'yes' or 'no' answer. They facilitate a discussion and help to establish a trusting, supportive environment that is conducive to reflection.

These types of questions allow many possible answers and often produce enlightening narrative. Moreover, they can be the key to asking deeper questions that are more challenging.

> **Appraiser**: 'How did you get on with your PDP last year?'
> **Appraisee**: 'I was quite pleased this year, despite being two partners short, I managed to attend a really helpful course on eye emergencies which I carried forward from last year'

Contrast this with the closed question below.

> **Appraiser**: 'Did you do the course on eye emergencies you carried forward from the last year?'

Apart from perhaps making the appraisee feel defensive, the second, more closed, question may not produce the information about the manpower deficiencies that the first, more open, question did.

> Further examples of open questions or phrases that lead to answers as though an open question had been asked:
> 'Tell me a bit more . . .'
> 'I was really interested to read about the audits you listed . . .would you like to tell me about one, perhaps one you found particularly useful?'
> 'Is there anything else you'd like to mention/raise/discuss?''

Closed questions

Such questions usually produce 'yes' or 'no' answers and could make the appraisee feel uncomfortable in many ways. For instance, they could suggest an expectation from the appraiser, which the appraisee cannot meet and lead to defensiveness.

> Further examples of closed questions:
> 'Have you undertaken a Basic Life Support Training this year?'
> 'How many audits have you personally undertaken?'

Closed questions are useful in the right place. A closed question can be a way to obtain specific information about a certain area.

For example, the first closed question in the box below gives the expected one-word response. The second closed question could give another closed answer or more of a story.

> **Appraiser:** 'How many partners do you aim for in your practice?'
> **Appraisee:** 'Three.'
> **Appraiser:** 'Do you mind whether they are part time?'
> **Appraisee:** 'No.'
> *or*
> **Appraisee:** 'Yes, my partners think we need fully committed clinicians. We don't want anyone who's going to be "swanning off" here and there and leaving us behind to do the real work.'

This demonstrates that classifications are pegs on which to hang description and discussion. The boundaries in questioning, as in many other areas, are not always clear and their use has to be flexible.

3 Reflecting

This technique is sometimes confused with 'mirroring', as described above. This is because reflecting is comparable to holding up a 'verbal mirror' to the appraisee and literally and accurately feeding back. This will give back (supportively) to the appraisee some of what they have said and some of the feelings the appraiser had picked up from their non-verbal language. It is a way of listening actively that enables both a non-judgemental attitude and an empathetic response to be demonstrated.

Staying with the example above, the appraisee has expressed a view that appears inflexible. Reflecting this statement is one way of exploring the views held.

> 'You say you all think you need fully committed clinicians. You seem angry with anyone who goes "swanning off"?'

It is constructive for the appraiser to keep as closely as possible to the appraisee's own words. However, adding a short question may help to move the appraisee's thinking a bit.

> 'You seem certain that only a colleague with a full-time clinical commitment will do. Have you had experience of a part-time colleague?'

Reflecting is a useful tool in the appraisal discussion. It is a method that encourages a peer relationship and assists the appraisee in recognising or accepting that they are thinking or feeling something that seems less acceptable. This may be about pride in achievement as well as more difficult emotions.

4 Challenging

Dogmatic statements can make a discussion falter. The appraiser may be inclined to ignore a rigid stance in order to avoid conflict. Yet that very thought might be paralysing the appraisee from actions that would allow them to achieve their aspirations.

Reflecting back the dogmatic statement as described above would be one way of challenging it without being confrontational.

It is sometimes helpful to challenge by asking what effect alternatives might have on the situation under discussion.

For the appraisee who believes that 'only full-time doctors are proper doctors', suggesting alternative scenarios might provoke an opening up of their approach.

> 'Have you thought about job sharing and how that might work in your practice?'
> 'What about an experienced colleague with family commitments such as looking after elderly parents? Do you think they might have something to offer your department?'

. . . or suggesting the unthinkable.

> 'What would be the consequences if you did not find someone to take on a "full-time clinical commitment"?'

The tone of voice used to ask these questions is important because the appraiser is aiming to encourage the appraisee to think in a way they may not have considered before. There should not be even a remote hint of the appraiser being judgemental. Instead, the appraiser needs to convey concern and support.

5 Getting back to safe ground

After exploring a difficult or sensitive issue, the appraiser has a responsibility to ensure that that section is closed before moving on. This technique is known as 'getting back on to safe ground'. The appraiser needs to check that the appraisee has something to move forward with, even if it simply means accepting that no change is possible at that particular time.

> 'Do you feel you have explored some acceptable ideas to help you move forward on this issue with your colleagues?'
> 'Are you feeling more settled about this issue, having discussed it, even though no solutions are apparent at this time?'

The appraiser may feel awkward checking verbally that the appraisee is back on safe ground. This process is vital to ensure that the appraisee is ready to concentrate on the next phase of the appraisal discussion. The appraisee will be particularly sensitive to cues at this stage and will pick up the appraiser's empathy and supportive non-verbal language.

6 Demonstrating empathy

Empathy has a specific meaning when used in the doctor–patient consultation. In the wider context, it is often used interchangeably with the word sympathy,[17] but they have distinct and separate meanings.

In the appraisal discussion, as with the medical consultation, empathy is used to communicate that the appraiser has an idea of how the appraisee is feeling and accepts it without judgement. This can often be done by non-verbal communication such as a brief touch on the arm or just being still. There is a fine line between empathising verbally and making the appraisee feel patronised. The sort of statement below is often thought of (mistakenly) as empathic. In fact, it takes the focus away from the appraisee, and might even prevent them from continuing with that particular train of thought.

> I know exactly how you feel . . . I felt exactly the same when I had my first complaint.

Demonstrating empathy does not mean that the appraisal discussion cannot be structured.

> It is good that you did not cancel your appraisal, with all the difficult things that have occurred since we arranged it. . . . Would it be helpful for us to try and decide together what you really need to discuss today?

Demonstrating empathy is a specialised tool in the appraiser's toolkit, which needs practice to be used effectively, but once mastered, can be a key to sensitive areas in the appraisal discussion.

7 Signposting

Signposting makes explicit the structure of the discussion to the appraisee. It is employed to mark the end of a section, the approach to a contentious topic or to suggest a break for thought. The appraiser, by sharing thinking and rationale for the next step of the discussion, shares the plan overtly with the appraisee.

It is particularly useful when the appraiser needs to move to a difficult area of the discussion. For example, an appraisee may have written something about feeling undervalued. To ease entry to this territory, the appraiser could acknowledge the trust required to raise this issue.

> Phrases that exemplify signposting:
>
> • 'I think it must have been quite difficult to raise your concerns about your attitude to drug addicts . . . it might be an idea to discuss that now . . .'

> - 'Would you like to describe the situation to me? That way we may be able to crystallise the issues and hopefully you might come up with some ideas about the way forward.'
> - 'We have been thinking and discussing your work in quite a lot of depth; shall we have a short break before we sort out your PDP? How long shall we take?'

If a suitable silence does not produce any comment at least the direction of discussion is clear.

8 Encouraging reflection

It is important that the appraisee is encouraged to reflect on statements, rather than the appraiser rushing to provide answers and solutions. The balance of talking between appraisee and appraiser should be heavily weighted (80:20) in favour of the appraisee.

While it has been stated in Chapter 3 that the appraiser is not a teacher, the appraiser may draw on adult education theory, as discussed in Chapter 2, to enable a truly reflective discussion.

9 Active listening

> Listening is being silent in an active way.
> **Morton Kelsey**[18]

Active listening is achieved by transmitting appropriate non-verbal messages to the appraisee, that the appraiser:

- is really interested in what the appraisee is saying
- wants to understand as fully as possible
- wants to help
- will not judge
- will be honest.

It is interesting to note that 'silent' and 'listen' are anagrams of each other.

10 Summarising

Summarising allows the appraiser to demonstrate an understanding of what the appraisee has said. It shows the appraisee that the appraiser has been listening attentively. It also means that the appraisee can correct, amplify or clarify anything important the appraiser seems to be unclear about. This needs to be done periodically during the appraisal discussion, and is particularly useful when moving from one area to the next.

11 Giving feedback

Feedback skills also need to be developed so that remarks by the appraiser are descriptive and non-judgemental. In reality, the entire appraisal discussion is a series of feedback sessions. All the communication skills described above need to be employed appropriately, but it is useful for the appraiser to have a variety of structures to draw on in order to give feedback that really helps the appraisee to develop.

There are some general principles that apply to giving feedback in any situation. The feedback needs to:

- focus on behaviour or action, not what the appraiser thinks
- give specific examples
- be non-judgemental
- be descriptive of what exists or has happened.

A more detailed list of 'the dos and don'ts of feedback' can be found in Chapter 11.

There are a plethora of feedback models, but two of the most commonly used which draw on the doctor–patient or teacher–learner situation will be discussed briefly here. They are:

- Pendleton[19]
- ALOBA (Agenda Led Outcome Based Analysis).[20]

Having stressed that the appraiser is not a teacher or doctor to the appraisee, it may seem inconsistent to suggest feedback models from medicine and teaching. However, these are useful tools.

In both feedback frameworks, the focus is on the appraisee, and this gives the appraiser a mechanism to facilitate reflection. However, the timing and flow of feedback between appraisee and appraiser are different in each method.

The Pendleton framework can be condensed into the steps in the box below.

- Appraisee invited to state positive aspects of area under discussion
- Appraiser comments or expands on positive aspects
- Appraisee invited to consider areas where things could have been done differently (care is used not to say better)
- Appraiser suggests areas that could be been done differently (not necessarily better)

The salient steps of ALOBA (modified to be applied to the appraisal discussion) are described below.

- Start with the appraisee's agenda: positive or negative
- Encourage appraisee to suggest ideas and solutions to move forward first
- Appraiser offers ideas that may move the appraisee's thinking to produce ideas and solutions
- If appraisee has focused on negative aspects the appraiser should point out positive achievements and progress
- Appraisee summarises action points before moving on to next topic

While Pendleton encourages the appraisee to think of all the positive achievements first, and a lot of effort is put into this, ALOBA, as the acronym suggests, encourages the appraisee to develop the agenda for discussion.

> Using Pendleton, the opening question might be:
>
> - 'Thinking about last year's PDP, could you please tell me what went particularly well?'
>
> Using ALOBA might result in an opening such as:
>
> - 'Is there anything you'd like us to specifically discuss in relation to last year's PDP?'

While the appraiser and appraisee are still settling into their relationship, appraisees can be particularly anxious about disclosing goals not met.

Their whole focus could be on what they have failed to deliver. The Pendleton approach, with its emphasis on positive first, could make the appraisee feel that the appraiser is not genuine or is being patronising. An open question allows the appraisee to raise issues that they think are important. The appraiser can discuss the important areas that the appraisee may have given less weight to when the appraisee's mind is less preoccupied with negative, insecure thoughts.

Pendleton's method is more overtly structured. The appraisee moves to areas that need developing only once the successes have been confirmed. The appraiser may use a question such as the one in the box below to introduce the topic of goals not reached.

> 'Now would you like to discuss anything that you wished had gone differently about last year's PDP?'

Using ALOBA, the appraisee is quite likely to have brought up goals that have not been achieved. Reasonable explanations or feeble excuses may be appropriately challenged by the appraiser. A discussion of what might be carried over to the next year's PDP might ensue, and the discussion should end on a positive note.

In the Pendleton model, the aim is also to finish on a positive note, leaving the appraisee with feedback that has been balanced and useful.

It is important to remember that the value of being made aware of a method of giving feedback is to provoke the appraiser to think about this topic. An appraiser does not have to choose one model and adhere to it. It is clear that there are elements that are common to giving feedback in any situation. The appraiser must give constructive feedback that will help an appraisee reflect and change behaviour.

In the above section, many skills and strategies have been explored to assist the appraiser in facilitating the appraisal discussion with a variety of appraisees in a diverse range of situations. As appraisers grow in confidence it is anticipated that they will develop their own styles, which can easily be adapted to suit the needs of individual appraisees.

Curtailing the appraisal

There are very rare occasions when an appraisal needs to be curtailed. Guidance from the Department of Health[7] requires the appraisal to be curtailed if the appraiser discovers previously unidentified poor performance, serious ill health or unprofessional behaviour. This is a very challenging situation for even the most experienced appraiser. The appraisee needs specific reasons for the curtailment of a process that could have involved hours of preparation. Honesty is best and the appraisers need to state who they will be discussing the situation with and how local procedures work.

The appraisee may become angry and could easily feel judged or discriminated against. The appraiser needs to be able to deal with these feelings.

It may be more appropriate to state that the appraisal has to be deferred until certain issues are clarified. That way the appraiser can create some breathing space. These difficult situations are also dealt with in Chapter 9.

Conclusion

The appraisal discussion should be a hugely privileged, worthwhile and developmental activity for the appraisee and appraiser alike. The appraiser needs highly developed communication skills to ensure the success of the appraisal discussion. These can be learnt and practised. The rewards if this is done are immense.

References

1   Silverman J, Kurtz S, Draper J. *Skills for Communicating with Patients*. 2nd ed. Oxford: Radcliffe Publishing; 2005.
2   Covey S. *The 7 habits of highly effective people*. London: Simon and Schuster; 1992.
3   Robinson P. *Meetings, Bloody Meetings*. York: Video Arts Ltd; 1976.
4   Ruusuvuori J. Looking means listening: coordinating displays of engagement in doctor–patient interaction. *Soc Sci Med*. 2001; **52**(7): 1093–108.
5   Gillen T. *The Appraisal Discussion*. London: Chartered Institute of Personnel and Development; 1995.
6   NHS Appraisal Toolkit. *Appraisal Toolkit Guidance*; 2003. www.appraisals.nhs.uk [accessed 19 August 2006].
7   Department of Health. *NHS Appraisal: guidance on appraisal for general practitioners working in the NHS*. London: DoH; 2002.
8   Department of Health. *Appraisal Forms for NHS Clinical Consultants*. 2001 [accessed 1 April 2006]. Available from: www.dh.gov.uk/assetRoot/04/03/46/24/04034624.doc
9   Neighbour R. *The Inner Apprentice*. Newbury: Petroc Press; 2000.
10 The University of Kentucky Centre for Learning Resources/WK Kellogg Foundation. Teaching Improvement Project System; 1975.
11 Grant J, Chambers E, Jackson G. *The Good CPD Guide: a practical guide to managed CPD*. Sutton: The Joint Centre for Education in Medicine; 1999.
12 Mehrabian A. *Silent Messages: implicit communication of emotions and attitudes*. 2nd ed. Belmont, CA: Wadsworth; 1981.
13 Birdwhistell RL. *Kinesics and Context*. Pennsylvania: University of Pennsylvania Press; 1970.

14 Pease A. *Body Language: how to read others' thoughts by their gestures.* London: Sheldon Press; 1984.

15 Bee F, Bee R. *Facilitation Skills.* London: Institute of Personnel and Development; 1998.

16 Mackay I. *Asking Questions.* 2nd ed. Brecon: Chartered Institute of Personnel Development Publishing; 1998.

17 Black D. Sympathy reconfigured: some reflections on sympathy, empathy and the discovery of values. *Int J Psychoanal.* 2004; **85**(3): 579–95.

18 Kelsey MT. *The Other Side of Silence: a guide to Christian meditation.* Mahwah, NJ: Paulist Press; 1976.

19 Pendleton D, Schofield T, Tate P, Havelock P. *The Consultation: an approach to learning and teaching.* Oxford: Oxford University Press; 1984.

20 Kurtz S, Silverman J, Draper J. *Teaching and Learning Communication Skills in Medicine.* 2nd ed. Oxford: Radcliffe Publishing; 2005.

Chapter 8

The paperwork for appraisal

This chapter aims to help the appraiser understand and use the appraisal paperwork effectively.

Form 4 and the personal development plan are important to provide evidence for the appraisal and to summarise the discussion and the development needs of the appraisee. They provide continuity between appraisals and are the tools for organisations to respond to needs identified in appraisal.

> We can lick gravity, but sometimes the paperwork is overwhelming.
>
> Wernher von Braun

Introduction

One of the few areas of appraisal for which there was national guidance from the beginning was the paperwork. The government laid out a series of forms, numbered 1 to 5 (or 6) based on the same headings as used in *Good Medical Practice* (Table 8.1).[1] The forms do vary slightly between primary and secondary care, in both headings and precise order, as laid out below. This has been discussed more fully in Chapter 2. These headings will be familiar to all doctors working within the NHS. They will already have encountered them in their own appraisals.

The structure of the forms is logical and the mapping onto *Good Medical Practice*, in Forms 3, 4 and 5, ensures that no significant area of professional life is missed. The same information may be provided in more than one section, but the guidance suggests that this is not necessary, and common sense should be used when the appraisee completes the paperwork.[2]

Table 8.1 Areas covered in appraisal for consultants and general practitioners

Consultants	General practitioners
Good medical care	Good clinical care
Maintaining good medical practice	Maintaining good medical practice
Working relationships with colleagues	Relationships with patients
Relations with patients	Working with colleagues
Teaching and training	Teaching and training
Probity	Probity
Health	Management activity
Management activity	Research
Research	Health

The paperwork varies across the UK, indeed some areas use an exclusively electronic format,[3] but the principles outlined in this chapter, although based on the original English system for appraisal, are broadly applicable to all formats.

A guide to the paperwork

The structure and content of Forms 1–3, which are completed by the appraisee before the appraisal discussion, are reviewed in Chapter 6. They, plus whatever supporting documentation the appraisee chooses to submit, form the basis for the appraiser's preparation.

This chapter will focus mainly on the facilitation of Form 4 and the personal development plan (PDP).

Form 4 summary document

The Form 4 is the summary of the appraisal discussion and is a vital component of appraisal. In most appraisal systems it comprises the written Form 4, with a separate tabulated PDP. It is the mirror of the appraisal and is the only written record of the content of the appraisal discussion. It pulls together key themes from the preparatory paperwork and the reflection by the appraisee.

The purpose of the written Form 4

- Summarises the appraisal discussion for the appraisee, providing a source for future reference.
- Summarises the appraisal discussion for the appraiser, although the appraiser does not keep a copy.
- Acts as a resource for producing the PDP; the two parts together being the true 'Form 4'.
- Provides structure to the discussion and ensures that each area within *Good Medical Practice* has been considered.
- Serves as the 'baton' that passes information from one year's appraisal to the next.
- Demonstrates that appraisal has taken place and may be used as part of the supporting evidence for revalidation.
- Demonstrates the appraisal has been documented to a certain standard. The presence (or absence) of a good Form 4 may be used as one of the tools to consider whether the appraiser is doing the appraising well. It is an indicator of the quality of the work of the appraiser.[4]
- Acts as a tool for the appraisal lead to collate learning and development needs for the organisation.

It is a real challenge for the appraiser to ensure that the document is written well and succinctly and yet also manages to effectively fulfil these purposes.

The form may be completed by the appraiser or the appraisee, but needs to have agreement and input from both parties. It may be completed at the time of appraisal discussion or may be developed by email after the discussion. What is vital is that the ownership and direction of the document, and its contents, are genuinely those of the appraisee.

What makes a good Form 4?

It is a real skill to be able to write, or enable the appraisee to write, good Form 4s. This can only be achieved by training, practice and ongoing discussion in appraiser support groups. Task and criteria have been suggested to develop the quality of the paperwork.[4,5]

A checklist for the appraiser to consider when reviewing the form is useful and is included in Chapter 11. This may be also be used by appraisal leads in reviewing the quality of Form 4s that they receive from appraisers.

Form 4 is an essential document. If it is well constructed it has the meat of the appraisal discussion laid out in an easily digestible form. It will contain all the significant positive and negative findings from the appraisal. It will include a consideration of the evidence for assertions that are made and of the action that needs to be taken as a result.

The good appraisal summary

Is legible

- No matter how good the content, it will not be useful if it cannot be read.
- Typed versions are generally preferable.
- Web-based systems such as the Welsh online appraisal or the NHS Appraisal Toolkit[6] achieve this naturally.

Is factually correct

- Information should be collated consistently and accurately.
- Co-signing by the appraiser and appraisee testifies to the Form 4 being factually correct.

Is relevant

- Form 4 is divided into sections under the *Good Medical Practice* headings.
- Comments should be relevant to these headings.
- There is no need to repeat comments that are relevant to more than one heading.

Is free of bias and prejudice

- Comments should be objective.

Acknowledges the appraisees achievements

- Significant positive aspects of a doctor's performance should be recorded in the summary.

Charts developmental progress

- Records development that has occurred.
- Shows how it has been achieved.

- Uses backward steps as recommendations for future action.
- May refer to the PDP if developmental progress is documented there.

Promotes the appraisee's professional development

- Constructively motivates the appraisee to improve.
- 'No action required' will not encourage the high flyer to improve.
- Admonishment is not usually motivational.

Is evidence based

- Evidence from the appraisee is necessary to make the appraisal meaningful and objective.
- Form 4 can be used to log the submission of appropriate evidence under each of the headings of *Good Medical Practice* and to make recommendations for future submissions.
- There are (currently) no requirements for specified evidence to be submitted for the appraisal. However, appraisees will want their appraisers to guide them in recording appropriate evidence that will be useful for revalidation.

Is challenging

- The appraisal is supportive and developmental but challenge is a valid tool to encourage development and the form should reflect this.

Is actionable

- Action points must be realistic and appropriate.
- Form 4 and the PDP are the baseline against which next year will be evaluated.
- Resource needs may be identified but some actions must be appropriate for the appraisee to be able to demonstrate year-on-year professional development.

Is acceptable to the appraisee

- Ownership by the appraisee is critical to the usefulness of these documents.
- Co-signature confirms the acceptability of the record of discussion, evaluation and recommendations to both parties.

The skilled appraiser is able to work with the appraisee to produce a summary of the appraisal discussion that is fit for the purposes described above and fulfils the criteria described. This challenging task requires considerable training, practice and commitment on the part of the appraiser. It is vitally important.

The personal development plan (PDP)

One outcome of appraisal is the PDP for the coming year. All appraisers need a good understanding of how to facilitate a PDP that will be useful and effective for the appraisee. Some development needs will not fit easily into an annual planning cycle and will need to be addressed over a longer period than one year.

The PDP is the key to the purpose of appraisal and should catalyse development for the appraisee. The plan should be personal to the appraisee, prioritised by the appraisee and appropriate for the appraisee.

Producing a PDP can be considered in terms of three main steps.

- Learning and developmental needs:
  - what are the appraisees' priorities for development in the context of their overall professional development?
- Continuing professional development (development activity):
  - how will appraisees best approach their needs in a way that is appropriate for them? (as discussed in Chapter 2).
- Recording development:
  - what will appraisees record to demonstrate that their needs have been addressed?

SMARTIES

It has been suggested that all the learning objectives in the PDP should be presented in terms of SMARTIES. These are a development of the idea of SMART objectives, an acronym that is so widely used that its origins are now obscure.

To be most useful to the individual and to the organisation a learning objective should be:

- **S**pecific
- **M**easurable
- **A**chievable
- **R**ealistic
- **T**ime-framed
- **I**nteresting
- **E**conomic
- **S**hared (also sometimes **S**cores, or **S**uccess).

Specific ideas have the sense of direction that will help an appraisee to know what to tackle and where to start.

Working out what an appraisee is trying to achieve and how to judge whether it has been accomplished can be done by building in the idea of a **measure** of success to that objective.

It is a key role of the appraiser to ensure that appraisees set themselves objectives that are **achievable**, by the appraisees in their unique circumstances, not by the appraiser.

Objectives must also be **realistic**. Many doctors will try to attempt too much and risk feeling that they have failed if they do not deliver on all that they planned.

An appropriate **timeframe** for the delivery of an objective should be explicit from the start. It would be unreasonable to leave finding a mentor to the week before the next appraisal, or to do a Certificate in Speciality Care in less than a year.

In addition, it may be helpful to check out with appraisees that their objectives are truly **interesting** to them. Whether the motivation is driven by personal or team needs, the specific objective must be framed so that the appraisee is motivated to complete the activity, reflecting the principles of adult education discussed in Chapter 2.

Targets must also be **economic** in terms of the time and effort required or they will fail to be achieved. An activity that requires a lot of resources will have to be particularly interesting or well rewarded to sustain the effort.

A final consideration is that the outcome of the learning must be a **success**. Such **scores** can usually be **shared** and it is worth planning how to do this. When the whole multiprofessional team benefits from the learning of one member, then the PDP has been particularly well designed.

It needs to be recognised that there are some individuals for whom a PDP is not a very useful tool.[7]

> Since the appraisal I have found other more pressing educational/clinical needs, both for my practice and myself and as such the plan in the appraisal had to be changed – leaving one feeling that the process is not flexible.

Some appraisees may prefer to see the big picture and do things more spontaneously than those who like to have a step-by-step plan. It is important for the appraiser to be aware of the appraisees' likely preferences and to help them to frame objectives in a way that is most useful for them as individuals. There can be a temptation to write a PDP that has SMARTIES objectives that are too easily achieved, being activities the appraisee has either already done or knows they will do easily without being challenged.

Using the Form 4 and PDP from one year should guide the activity that a doctor undertakes in the next. There should be room for adaptation and opportunistic

Table 8.2 An example PDP objective for opportunistic learning

What development needs have I?	How will I address them?	Date by which I plan to achieve the development goal	Outcome	Completed
Explain the need	Explain how you will take action, and what resources you will need	The date agreed with your appraiser for achieving the development goal	How will your practice change as a result of the development activity?	Agreement from your appraiser that the development need has been met
To capture examples of opportunistic learning and the reflection arising	Devise a system to record reflective notes on learning that takes place in an unplanned way	System in place by 4 weeks, used all year with at least one record per month	There will be a better record of opportunistic learning and of my reflection at the time which will aid me in identifying patterns about what I should target	

learning, as and when something comes up during the year. Some doctors find it hard to decide in advance what they wish to cover and may need to write into their PDP an objective that allows flexibility throughout the year to pursue avenues of interest arising out of cases that arise, articles they may read or events that come up. An example is given in Table 8.2.

Evaluating Form 4 and the PDP

If these two documents are important as appraisal outputs, it is imperative that they are well written and facilitated. While the forms should be appraisee-owned in terms of content, skilled appraisers can facilitate much better documentation than the appraisee might produce alone.

Appraiser support groups should use anonymised forms, or forms written for training purposes, to reflect on how the paperwork may be improved.

Form 5 for secondary care

Form 5 for secondary care clinicians is very different from the Form 5 for GPs. It has a stated aim of informing the job plan review and so asks the appraisee to describe their effectiveness on a personal level and within the employing organisation. It specifically asks the appraiser to prepare a workload summary with the appraisee.

Although it asks for the appraisees' identification of the resources needed to improve personal effectiveness, the bulk of the documentation and reflection is targeted at service-related objectives and deriving any proposed changes to the job plan. It may be used to introduce a performance management element to the appraisal process.

Detailed confidential account of appraisal discussion

There is a further form that is similar to Form 4. It was intended to be used as a further entirely confidential record of the appraisal discussion. Confusingly, it is numbered Form 5 when used by GPs and Form 6 when used by consultants.

In practice, it is very rarely used in most appraisal systems. The guidance notes are the same for both primary and secondary care. They emphasise the optional nature of the framework for keeping a fuller account of the appraisal discussion and suggest that its use would be to inform the next appraisal round. The notes underline the fact that this form is confidential and not intended to form part of the documentation that is shared after the appraisal.

It is also made clear that this form is not to be used to record details of poor performance that might affect patient care or serious concerns about colleagues that should be the subject of action.

Because completion is not obligatory, anecdotally, very few appraisals result in the production of this type of Form 5 or 6. Of course, by its very nature this form would be kept confidential so it is hard to be sure of the truth of this assertion.

The signing-off process

The sign off, which indicates the acceptance and completion of the Form 4 and PDP, is an important part of the appraisal paperwork. It usually marks the end of the appraisal and has a satisfying sense of achievement to it.

Some appraisees have other types of appraisal in relation to other roles that they may undertake (as discussed in Chapter 9) and these can be recorded here, with the details of the third-party appraisers who contributed.

Evaluation forms

Although they are vital for the quality assurance of the appraisers' performance, there are no standard evaluation forms. Suggestions for best practice are discussed in more detail in Chapter 10 and examples are included in Chapter 12.

Conclusion

The paperwork for appraisal is familiar to all doctors working in the NHS because they have used it in their own appraisals. There are differences between the paperwork for primary and secondary care and between the four nations of the UK. There are also some special adaptations for doctors in complex situations. However, the themes remain constant.

If well done, the summary of the appraisal discussion and the PDP will ensure that appraisal is not a stand-alone activity. It will transform the development of the individual and inform the development of the organisation.

References

1 General Medical Council. *Good Medical Practice*. 3rd ed. London: GMC; 2001.
2 Department of Health. *NHS Appraisal: guidance on appraisal for general practitioners working in the NHS*. London: DoH; 2002.
3 GP Appraisal and CPD Unit. *GP Appraisal in Wales: annual report 2004/2005*. Cardiff: Cardiff University School of Postgraduate Medical and Dental education; 2005.
4 Jelley D. *Writing a Good Form 4 – why bother?* Newcastle: Northern Deanery; 2005.
5 Rughani A. *GP Appraisal Forms 3 and 4: providing guidance and setting standards*. Sheffield: South Yorkshire and South Humber Deanery; 2003.
6 NHS Appraisal Toolkit. *Appraisal Toolkit Guidance*; 2003. www.appraisals.nhs.uk [accessed 19 August 2006].
7 Hunt W. *Northamptonshire Heartlands Annual Appraisal Report*. Northampton: Northamptonshire Heartlands PCT; 2004.

Chapter 9

Complex appraisal situations

This chapter considers how the appraiser should approach different groups of doctors. Alternative models of appraisal that may be required in complex situations are reviewed.

> All that is valuable in human society depends upon the opportunity for development accorded the individual.
>
> **Albert Einstein (1879–1955)**

Introduction

An increasing number of doctors are diversifying their activities and undertaking several roles alongside their clinical work. Some of them work in an environment that does not fit neatly into mainstream NHS practice.

For most doctors, the appropriate appraiser is clear. A GP appraises a GP. However, there may be discussion as to whether general surgeons are fully equipped to appraise gynaecologists, even though both come from a surgical background. In the extreme, a paediatric cardiothoracic surgeon may feel that only a colleague in the same subspeciality can undertake an appropriate appraisal with him.

From the appraiser's perspective, each appraisal is an experience that requires effort, thought and preparation. However, there are some situations outside the routine experience of the appraiser, which might diminish the effectiveness of the appraisal. This may be because they are unfamiliar, occur rarely and are less well rehearsed. There may be particular considerations that must be addressed to create the environment for a successful appraisal.

Appraisees in the context of the team

Appraisal processes, as they have been developed so far, are designed to focus on individual clinicians. Doctors often present evidence that relates to the whole team. It is common to find that the constraints that prevent a doctor developing and delivering good care, relate to systems within the organisation,[1] which the appraisee may feel powerless to address. During the appraisal discussion, appraisers need the right skills to facilitate the appraisee in focusing on their own personal activity within the team. They also need to challenge the appraisee to reflect on whether blocks to development are real or perceived.

It is important that the team as a whole develops an action plan to improve the services and care delivered to patients. In primary care, some forward-thinking practices combine this action plan with the development plans gleaned from the appraisal of individuals within the team to form a practice professional development plan (PPDP).[2,3] This form of planning is enhanced by including all members of the team, whatever their professional background.

Appropriately used, the PPDP allows for individual PDPs to be addressed, while realising the developmental objectives of the organisation or team.

Doctors like Maria

Delivering effective appraisal for 'doctors like Maria'[4] requires careful organisation. It is worth considering some examples of doctors (Table 9.1) for whom particular considerations apply in appraisal.

The list of doctors below is illustrative rather than comprehensive.

Doctors with particular training and support needs

- Doctors in training.
- Returners.
- Retained doctors and others with minimal clinical commitment.
- Locums and sessional doctors.
- Out-of-hours (OOH) doctors (UK trained or based but isolated due to the nature of their work).
- Out-of-hours (OOH) doctors (those who fly in from abroad).
- European Union (EU) doctors.
- Refugee doctors.

Private practice

- Doctors undertaking private work alongside their NHS posts.
- Doctors who provide services entirely privately.

Portfolio clinicians

- A specialised clinical role (e.g. general practitioners with a special interest (GPwSIs).
- An additional research or academic role.
- Medical educators (e.g. trainers, clinical tutors, GP tutors, undergraduate teachers).
- Management roles (e.g. medical directors, clinical governance leads).
- Appraisers and appraisal leads.
- Combining two professions (architecture and medicine).

Doctors who work in unusual environments

- Prison doctors.
- Police surgeons.
- Doctors in the armed forces.

Doctors in various sorts of difficulty

- Poorly performing doctors.
- Sick doctors.

Table 9.1 Appraisees with particular challenges

Doctor	Issues the appraiser needs to be aware of
Doctors with particular training and support needs	
Doctors in training	Under continual summative assessment (including RITAs)
Returners to general practice	Need to acquire externally defined competencies
	Developing reflective skills
	Learning about appraisal
	Need educational and clinical supervisors as well as an appraiser
	Changing jobs frequently may make it difficult to collect evidence
Retained doctors and others with minimal clinical commitment	Small number of hours worked
	Domestic and other competing pressures
	Less opportunity for experiential learning
	Less opportunity to be involved in the team
	Difficulty collecting information about individual practice
Locums and sessional doctors	Difficulty collecting information about individual practice
	Lack of support mechanisms
	Lack of security of employment
	No protected holiday and sick leave
	Insecurity may breed low self-esteem
Out-of-hours (OOH) doctors (UK trained)	Professionally isolated due to working patterns
	Access to educational meetings limited
	Difficulty collecting information about individual practice
	Specialised caseload
	Difficult working environments
Out-of-hours (OOH) doctors (those who fly in from abroad)	Professionally isolated due to working patterns
	Access to educational meetings limited
	Difficulty collecting information about individual practice
	Specialised caseload
	Difficult working environments
	Mainly working in other country's regulatory system
	Potential for language problems
	May not understand UK appraisal system
	Limited knowledge of NHS
European Union (EU) doctors[5]	Unrestricted legal right to work
	Potential for language problems
	Potential cross-cultural problems
	Different training background
	Awareness of support and induction programmes (*see* Chapter 11)
Refugee doctors	Change of status in society compared with country of origin
	Potential for language problems
	Sensitivity to different nuances of non-verbal communication
	Understanding of different medical cultural backgrounds[6]
	Different training background
	May have experienced significant trauma
	Awareness of support and induction programmes (*see* Chapter 11)[7]
Private practice	
Doctors undertaking private work alongside their NHS posts	Explicitly included in normal NHS appraisal process for NHS consultant
	Potentially poor systems for data collection
	Potentially competing commitments and time pressures
Doctors who provide services entirely privately	No statutory requirement under NHS appraisal scheme
	May have difficulty in accessing appraisers
	May be subject to private providers appraisal processes

Table 9.1 (*cont.*)

Doctor	Issues the appraiser needs to be aware of
Portfolio clinicians	
A specialised clinical role (e.g. general practitioners with a special interest)	Potentially competing commitments and time pressures
	Separate roles may require separate appraisals
	Complexity of different roles
An additional research or academic role	Erosion of boundaries between roles and home life
	Potential for over commitment
Medical educators (e.g. trainers, clinical tutors, GP tutors, undergraduate teachers)	Accountable to multiple employers
Management roles (e.g. medical directors, clinical governance leads)	
Appraisers and appraisal leads	
Combining two professions (e.g. architecture and medicine)	
Doctors who work in unusual environments	
Prison doctors[8,9]	Work in more managed environment
Police surgeons	More hierarchical structures
Doctors in the armed forces	May have ethical conflicts to resolve
	May have separate performance management procedures
	Specialised caseload
	Particular issues around confidentiality in specialised environments

Appraisees with particular challenges

The appraiser needs to have an understanding of the unique issues that may impinge on the development of any doctor in order to prepare appropriately for the appraisal interview.

The doctors above are worthy of particular consideration. Signposting to developmental tools and resources may be especially relevant to these groups.

It is the responsibility of the organisation employing the appraiser to ensure that the appraiser has access to training for appraising these groups of doctors. However, an appraiser who opts to appraise them also has a professional responsibility to acquire the necessary skills.

Good Medical Practice[10] provides a good framework on which to base the analysis of the complexity of appraisal in this group of clinicians.

The particular appraisal issues that are pertinent to the appraisal of doctors like Maria are now explored.

All doctors have particular considerations and the table is not exhaustive. The groups mentioned have been used to illustrate approaches that appraisers should use in order to prepare themselves effectively. Like all doctors, these appraisees need to feel valued and respected.

Declining an appraisee

Having reflected on the issues surrounding an appraisal, appraisers must have the courage to decline an appraisee. If they have serious doubts about their ability or willingness to carry out an appraisal they must be prepared to give honest reasons for their decision.

> Dr Senior, I am delighted that you have asked me to undertake your appraisal. I am sorry I will have to decline. You are a senior GP who works in many areas in which I have no experience. I am still building up my skills as an appraiser and do not feel I am the best member of the appraisal team to provide you with an effective appraisal. Would you like to me to ask the appraisal lead to match you with someone else or would you prefer to make the arrangements yourself?

This may be one of the most difficult situations an appraiser has to deal with and it needs to be done sensitively.

Doctors in various sorts of difficulty

Poorly performing doctors

As stated previously, poor performance should not become apparent *de novo* during an appraisal, and if it does, the guidance is clear that the appraisal should be stopped and steps taken to set poor performance procedures in motion.[6,11]

However, a doctor whose performance has been found to be a risk to patients could well benefit from an appraisal. Does the doctor accept the findings? While it will be complicated to facilitate the doctor to reflect constructively on a situation that could be threatening his livelihood, if successful, appraisal could be rewarding. The poorly performing doctor may have a formal 'educational prescription' of learning needs to address, but their behaviour may not change, or any change that does occur may not be maintained, unless they own their development and their PDP.

It is important to stress that a doctor who is undergoing poor performance procedures needs multifaceted support, of which appraisal is only one part. A mentor and teacher may well also be needed.

Sick doctors

Dr Clive Froggatt (former heroin addict and GP advisor to the Government) said at the conference 'Doctors and their health: who heals the healers?' at St George's Hospital Medical School in London in 1996:

> Doctors do not ask for help for themselves, only for others. As a patient, I found asking for personal help, let alone accepting it, incredibly difficult. By then I was, in my own view, utterly unworthy.[8]

There is little evidence that this has changed, as doctors worry that illness will be

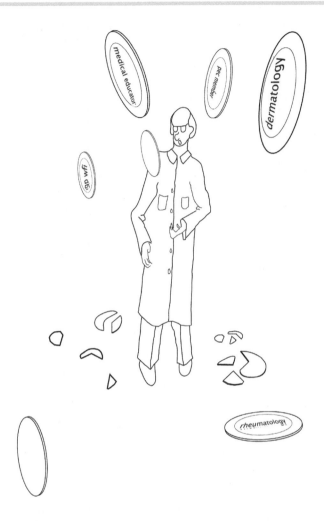

seen as a sign of weakness. The fear is that they will lose their job and all that goes with it.

At the same conference, Dr Hamid Ghodse, professor of psychiatry of addictive behaviour at St George's Hospital Medical School, London, said:

> The most successful outcome of treatment of a doctor-patient occurs when a sick doctor is approached in a friendly fashion by a fellow professional with an attitude of aid and support, rather than when the sick doctor is subjected to criticism or punishment for misconduct.

A sick doctor may find that the atmosphere in an appraisal is such that they feel comfortable, or even compelled, to disclose their illness. If the appraiser feels patient safety is at risk the appraisal must be stopped as discussed in Chapter 5.

The appraiser's job is to encourage the appraisee to agree to seek help and to disclose the illness to those who need to know, while not slipping imperceptibly into the 'doctor' role.

Table 9.2 Personal development plan to consider a health issue

What development needs do I have?	How will I address them?	Date by which I plan to achieve the development goal	Outcome	Completed
Explain the need	Explain how you will take action, and what resources you will need	The date agreed with your appraiser for achieving the development goal	How will your practice change as a result of the development activity?	Agreement from your appraiser that the development need has been met
To confront and manage my health issue, quantifying my deafness and identifying appropriate safeguards for patients	To see my GP, have audiometry and investigate use of electronic stethoscopes if necessary to do so	As soon as possible	I will have minimised the risk to my health and work and safeguarded patient care	

If it is clear that patients are not at risk but that there is a health issue, the appraiser needs to help the appraisee to crystallise the issues, discuss the implications (possibly unfounded fears) and negotiate a way forward. In this case an entry in the PDP might well be appropriate, as outlined in Table 9.2. The appraiser also needs to know about some of the support services available and some of these are considered in Chapter 11.

Alternative appraisal models

The importance of considering any unusual circumstances when preparing for the appraisal has been discussed. It is now appropriate to consider the systems necessary to support both the appraiser and appraisee in carrying out this task.

Current appraisal processes need to be examined to assess whether they can be adapted for all types of appraisee. If organisations and institutions were to collaborate more, it would avoid some doctors spending a disproportionate percentage of their working time being appraised.

We discuss five appraisal models below, some of which are currently being used. One or more model may suit a particular circumstance. They are presented as a basis for discussion and to give appraisal leads and others involved in the organisation of doctors' appraisals food for thought as they refine their appraisal systems.

A robust and effective appraisal should be the outcome whatever the process employed.

The five models considered are:

- joint appraisals
- appraisals with a specialist appraiser
- non-peer appraisals

- variable appraisal cycles
- external and internal appraisals.

In proposing alternative models of appraisal it important that the responsible organisation ensures the quality of the appraisal and its supporting systems. Communication channels need to be very clear, especially if appraisals are undertaken across organisations.

Joint appraisals

The common factor for doctors who may require a joint appraisal is that they undertake more than one role, each role being significant enough to require an appraisal. For example:

- doctors combining a secondary and primary care role
- doctors who hold academic posts
- GPwSIs.

The proposal recognises that each organisation requires the doctor to have a yearly appraisal. The appraisers in those organisations may feel they do not have the skills to appraise certain aspects of the appraisee's work.

Joint appraisals for doctors combining a secondary and primary care role

A part-time consultant psychiatrist, who also works as a sessional GP, currently has two appraisals, a GP appraisal and a mental health trust appraisal. He said to his GP appraiser:

> Would it not make more sense if you got together with my other appraiser? She does not have an overall picture of my work and neither do you. At least you should read both sets of paperwork.

This encapsulates the issue for such doctors. It may be that in some areas, the situation has been resolved. If not, there is practical experience of a model for the joint appraisal of academic doctors, which is described below.

Joint appraisals for doctors who hold academic posts

A GP also holds a substantive academic post with a London teaching hospital. The academic appraisal needs to be quite robust and focused. His work as a GP partner is undertaken in a busy GP practice.

Joint appraisal for academic clinical consultants outlined above began in the round for 2002–03.[9] A clinical appraiser and an academic appraiser co-facilitating the appraisal has been found to be a workable solution.

As the consultant Forms 1–3 and Form 5 (consultant version) are more comprehensive, and encompass all the headings the of GP forms, it would be logical to use suitably adapted consultant forms to prepare for the appraisal in both secondary and primary care. The Form 4 and PDP are common to both systems.

Chapter 6 has laid out the preparation necessary for every appraisal. For a joint appraisal, it is just as essential for both appraisers to prepare for the appraisal discussion. The co-appraisers need to formulate a plan for undertaking the appraisal. This can be done by telephone, although some may prefer a brief meeting immediately prior to the appraisal. For example, the clinical appraiser could 'lead' with the academic appraiser contributing/taking over when research, teaching and other academic issues arise.

At the beginning of the discussion, the proposed structure for the appraisal agreed between the appraisers needs to be negotiated with the appraisee. The co-appraisers need to work as a team. Although the agreed structure may not be strictly adhered to, it is helpful to give an overall direction to the appraisal discussion.

The duration of the appraisal discussion generally varies. These appraisals were reported as long, but within the range described by single appraisers (2–5 hours).[12]

The main benefit was the PDP. The appraisee felt that because it was the result of an in-depth discussion about all areas of his work, it reflected a more balanced plan than if only one appraiser had undertaken the appraisal.

> 'We have not evaluated them formally. From speaking to other colleagues involved in the process, I can say that we feel they are more effective than individual academic and clinical appraisals. Personally, I have found these appraisals useful and prefer the efficiency of joint ones.'

Both appraiser and the appraisee need to agree whether the discussion under the consultant Form 5 (Personal and organisational effectiveness) should occur at the joint appraisal, as this usually relates to the academic activities only. However, it may be interesting and developmental for the clinical appraiser to see how the performance review is carried out. Many would reasonably argue that both appraisers should complete the whole appraisal at the same time. On the other hand, deferring this part may help with time management and reduce the risk of the joint appraisal becoming too long, with a consequent loss of focus and interest.

Joint appraisal for general practitioners with a special interest (GPwSIs)

The Royal College of General Practitioners (RCGP) defines a GPwSI as:

> A GP with additional training and experience in a specific clinical area who takes referrals for assessment/treatment of patients outside GMS/ PMS that may otherwise have been referred directly to a secondary care consultant, or who provides an enhanced service for particular conditions or patient groups. GPwSIs are generally appointed to meet the needs of a single PCT or group of PCTs, and typically undertake two sessions per week in their specialty.[13]

GPwSIs often spend the majority of their time being a GP, using their art as a generalist, complemented by their special interests. It is accepted that a clinician needs an appraisal that covers each part of their work. The joint appraisal model can be applied to this group of doctors, to achieve an efficient use of time and resources while serving the needs of the appraisee.

In many situations where doctors undertake more than one role, one of their roles is likely be formally performance managed. The timing of the performance review process, relative to appraisal would need to be negotiated by all parties.[14]

This proposal and others are discussed by Gerada.[15]

The pros and cons of joint appraisal models

If suitable co-appraisers undertake the appraisal together, there are benefits for the appraisee.

Arguments for joint appraisal

- It allows the appraisee to reflect on the areas of overlap in two separate areas of work. The strengths they bring to each job can be emphasised and this is a way to enhance their practice in both areas without extra effort.
- In addressing areas of weakness in one role, they might glean ideas that would work in the other.
- The main benefit is production of a SMARTIES PDP (*see* Chapter 8).
- The PDP could be balanced over time. With both appraisers agreeing the PDP, the appraisee will have greater opportunity to formulate a PDP that has taken account of all their work in equal depth.
- A copy of the Form 4 and PDP needs to go to each organisation to inform their organisational development plans.
- It is a more efficient use of time, particularly for the appraisee.

Arguments against joint appraisal

- They are more difficult to organise (three busy people to meet).
- Each appraiser has a lot more reading to do. As the system develops it may be possible to send relevant supporting evidence to each appraiser, while both appraisers receive the Forms 1, 2 and 3.
- In trying to balance the appraisee's PDP, the appraisers may find it difficult to work out how much effort needs to be put into each area. However, those who undertake joint roles generally already appreciate that they are accompanied by a need for an increased range of competencies. Joint appraisals should not be seen as a means of getting a less onerous PDP.

Appraisals with a specialist appraiser

Another approach might be to develop a group of appraisers from a similar background with special interests.

Specialist appraisal of GPwSIs

An appraisal system for GPwSIs in respiratory medicine that uses this model has been proposed.[16] This proposal involves collaboration between national, local secondary and primary care bodies involved in respiratory care to develop and support appraisers with special interests in this field. They acknowledge the need for variability of appraisal dependent on the experience of the GPwSI and a focus on the development of a quality-assured national system that has the confidence of patients, doctors and NHS managers.

This model could form the basis for developing specialist appraisers in many fields, but further work needs to be done to demonstrate that the outcomes of such appraisals and the support needed to address the identified learning needs are worth the resources invested.

Clinicians with such similar backgrounds and interests may be at increased risk of colluding with each other. On the other hand, it could be argued that collusion could occur in any appraisal situation, and that the benefit gained from having an appraiser who would more readily understand the goals of the appraisee outweighs the theoretically negative aspect.

The conversation below demonstrates the risk of collusion in this context.

> **Appraisee:** 'I am concerned about the amount of time I spend doing clinical work . . . one session a week . . . is that sufficient to keep my skills up?'
>
> **Appraiser:** I don't know why you should feel that. Medicine's like riding a bike. With so much experience behind you, you should be all right. Anyway I am doing about the same amount!'

If this idea were to be developed, and taking into account the possible numbers of doctors who might benefit, the organisation would need to be on a large scale.

The deaneries might be the reasonable body to facilitate the development of such appraisers. Collaboration across deaneries, which already exists, could then allow clinicians with a variety of specialised interests to have access to appraisers with a similar background. Specialist appraisers or their appraisees might need to travel longer distances to secure an appropriate match.

The process being developed needs to be underpinned by a robust system for feedback and audit to ensure that the goal of effective appraisal is always met.

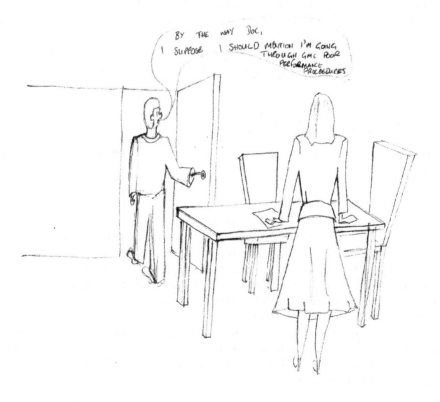

Non-peer appraisals

This is a thorny issue. In some ways it is the antithesis of the idea of specialist appraisers described above. Appraisal for doctors was set up as peer appraisal and it has evolved into a system where the term 'peer' has been interpreted to mean that GPs appraise GPs and consultants appraise consultants. However, it has been suggested that any well-trained appraiser, even those who are not doctors, may be suitable to appraise doctors.

If appraisal is a truly formative and developmental process whereby the appraisee is facilitated to reflect on various aspects of their work, should an experienced facilitator not be able to do this regardless of background?

This model is likely to raise significant protest from all the advocates of specialist appraisers and peer appraisal. The main concern is the ability of a non-doctor, or even more particularly, a non-clinician, to create the mutual trust and understanding to facilitate a truly open discussion. At its inception, appraisal was perceived by some doctors as threatening[17] and the threat was reduced by using a peer appraisal model.

There is a concern that using non-peer appraisers might result in less highly skilled appraisers. They cannot draw on the consultation skills that doctors have already learned. Many would see the appointment of non-peers as a cost-cutting exercise. There is the added valid objection that non-doctors do not have the knowledge to undertake appraisal of the 'Good clinical care' section.

If this idea were to be seriously considered, it would need a lot of thought so that the right 'non-peers' were appointed to appraise doctors. It should not be dismissed out of hand. There are individuals, particularly some nurses with educational experience, who would be able to demonstrate all the necessary competencies to become very skilful appraisers.

Variable appraisal cycles

For some appraisees none of the proposed models may meet their needs. Some individuals have too many roles to make a single joint or specialist appraisal possible. Variable appraisal cycles are a further option.

At the moment the guidance from the Department of Health[18] is that NHS clinicians should have an annual appraisal. If this is applied rigidly to every role a portfolio clinician has, it can be a resource-intensive process. This is particularly so if all aspects of a clinician's work are to be appraised, and several appraisals are deemed necessary. What if different aspects of a clinician's professional activity were appraised over the course of an appraisal cycle?

For example a GP with a long-standing clinical assistant role in ophthalmology has recently studied to become a GPwSI in sexual health and taken on a management role at the primary care organisation.

- Does this GP need four separate appraisals every year?
- Is there a way of combining one or more into joint appraisals?
- Do all roles really require an annual appraisal in depth?
- Can some be covered on a less frequent basis, perhaps once or twice in a five-year cycle?

- Is there enough flexibility in the structure of the main clinical appraisal to cover all roles?

The appraisee would need to discuss their individual appraisal cycle with all the different organisations they work for and, particularly, the trust with overall responsibility for the doctor's appraisal. This discussion could be facilitated by the appraisal lead of the responsible trust. All parties would have to agree the documentation that should be used for the pre-appraisal preparation and what would be shared post-appraisal. Appraisal cycles would need to be tailored to meet the needs of the individual appraisee. This would enable the appraisee to work intensively on each aspect of their work, while keeping tabs on the less-pressing learning needs at any given time.

This model is open to serious criticism on at least two counts. First, the benefit of two consecutive appraisals by the same appraiser may be lost. A difficult issue may have been raised last time and be conveniently ignored by the appraisee. The rapport with a different appraiser will not spring fully formed, as it often does on a return visit with the same appraiser.

There is also the argument that those who have several roles are somehow favoured, as they will not be required to produce the same rigorous core evidence for a standard appraisal every year.

There are real pragmatic advantages to this model allowing an efficient use of appraisal resources.

External and internal appraisals

Systems of appraisal can be classified as external and internal. External systems are those in which the appraiser is not a close colleague of the appraisee. In some cases they may not even have met prior to the appraisal. Internal appraisals are those where the appraiser and appraisee have a year-round professional relationship.

In the main, secondary care appraisals are internal. Appraisal of consultants is often by the clinical director of the department, this activity being part of the job description. General practice on the other hand has generally adopted external appraisal.

Where internal appraisal occurred before formal appraisal started, two studies,[19,20] explored the pros and cons of internal peer appraisal. A recent study[21] sought to determine the potential strengths and weaknesses of internal and external appraisals in delivering appraisal.

These studies demonstrated that both internal and external appraisals can provide appraisees with good or bad experiences. Appraisees reported a good appraisal if their goals were met and this was facilitated by the appraisees being able to choose their appraiser.

When the appraisers are from the same team, for example the same GP practice, as the appraisees, there may be a much more intimate knowledge of the appraisee's professional situation. Appraisal arrangements are easier to make and the logistics of access to supporting evidence is easier.

The risk for collusion is particularly present in this model. If one of the doctors has other roles, it may be appropriate for them to have their appraisal using one of the other models discussed above.

In matching appraisees, in this or any other appraisal process, it is the skills of the appraiser that are paramount. In this model it would also be possible for pairs of appraisers to co-appraise one another. This would be efficient in terms of resources and might bring greater depths to the discussion but might appear even more collusive.

The appraisee needs a system to access an appraiser who has the appropriate skills to provide the appraisal that best helps the appraisee to develop.

The appraisal system should have flexibility to meet the developmental needs of the appraisee and be fully quality assured.

Conclusion

It is now more than three years since universal annual appraisal of doctors in the NHS was introduced. This chapter contains ideas to provoke those involved in appraisal to think about the processes that have evolved and how they might develop further. It seems clear that some alternative appraisal models will be needed, tailored to the needs of the many types of extraordinary appraisee.

References

1 Cox J, King J, Hutchinson A, McAvoy P. *Understanding Doctors' Performance*. Oxford: Radcliffe Publishing; 2006.
2 Middleton J. A reflective log linked to personal development plans (PDPs) and the practice development plan (PPDP). *Educ Prim Care*. 2005; 16: 593–7.
3 Wilcock P, Campion-Smith C, Elston S. *Practice Professional Development Planning: a guide for primary care*. Oxford: Radcliffe Medical Press; 2003.
4 Martin D, Harrison P, Joesbury H, Wilson R. *Appraisal for GPs*. Sheffield: University of Sheffield School of Health and Related Research (ScHARR); 2001.
5 Ballard K, Laurence P. An induction programme for European general practitioners coming to work in England: development and evaluation. *Educ Prim Care*. 2004; 15(4): 584–95.
6 Department of Health. *NHS Appraisal: appraisal for consultants working in the NHS*. London: DoH; 1999.
7 Trewby PN. '. . . a stranger in a strange land': the plight of refugee doctors in UK clinical medicine. *J R Coll Phys*. 2005; 5(4): 317–19.
8 Wise J. Sick doctors need special treatment. *BMJ*. 1996; 313(7060): 771.
9 Department of Health. Appraisal for academic clinical consultants. 2002 [accessed 26 April 2006]. Available from: www.dh.gov.uk/PolicyAndGuidance/HumanResources AndTraining/LearningAndPersonalDevelopment/Appraisals/AppraisalsArticle/fs/ en?CONTENT_ID=4052035&chk=QQym5X
10 General Medical Council. *Good Medical Practice*. 2001 [accessed 14 April 2006]. Available from: www.gmc-uk.org/guidance/good_medical_practice/index.asp
11 Department of Health. *NHS Appraisal: guidance on appraisal for general practitioners working in the NHS*. London: DoH; 2002.
12 Central Cheshire Primary Care Trust. *GP Appraisal: annual report 2004*. Nantwich: CCPCT; 2004.
13 Royal College of General Practitioners. *Being a General Practitioner*. London: RCGP; 2006.
14 Birch K. *Developing Practitioners with Special Interest (PwSI) Services: managing the risks* [accessed 24 April 2006]. Available from: www.natpact.nhs.uk/uploads/PWSIManaging Risks.doc

15 Gerada C. *Appraisal, Revalidation of General Practitioners with Special Clinical Interest GPwSIs.* 2003 [accessed 22 April 2006]. Available from: www.appraisalsupport.nhs. uk/files2/12092004161143gpwsi.pdf

16 Holmes S, Gruffydd-Jones K. A proposal for the annual appraisal of, and developmental support for, general practitioners with a specialist interest (GPwSIs) in respiratory medicine. *Prim Care Resp J.* 2005; **14**(3): 161–5.

17 Lewis M, Elwyn G, Wood F. Appraisal of family doctors: an evaluation study. *Br J Gen Pract.* 2003; **53**(491): 454–60.

18 Department of Health. *Appraisals.* 1999 [accessed 26 April 2006]. Available from: www.dh.gov.uk/PolicyAndGuidance/HumanResourcesAndTraining/LearningAnd PersonalDevelopment/Appraisals/AppraisalsArticle/fs/en?CONTENT_ID=4080275 &chk=zoQbRx

19 Jelley D, van Zwanenberg T. Peer appraisal in general practice: a descriptive study in the Northern Deanery. *Educ Gen Pract.* 2000; **11**: 281–7.

20 Jelley D, van Zwanenberg T. Practice-based peer appraisal in general practice: an idea whose time has come? *Educ Prim Care.* 2003; **14**: 329-37.

21 Adams R, Illing J, Jelley D, Walker C, van Zwanenberg T. The critical success factors in internal and external appraisal. *Educ Prim Care.* 2006; **17**(6): 607–16.

Chapter 10

Quality assurance of appraisal: doing it well

This chapter considers how appraisers and those organising appraisal can work together to ensure that appraisals are done well. This is not an 'optional extra' but a responsibility incumbent on all involved in carrying out appraisals for doctors.

Quality means doing it right when no one is looking.
Henry Ford

Introduction

Quality assurance is one of those phrases that can strike fear and misgivings into some doctors. There is certainly a view that the NHS can be over-managed at times and some doctors may feel that they are best left to get on with the job themselves.

A well-designed quality assurance system does not seek to count and process endless paperwork. It aims to look at the whole appraisal process and consider whether it delivers high-quality appraisals that will effectively support doctors and lead to better patient care. Quality assurance should ensure that the appraisal process is carried out well and, equally importantly, should lay out guidance and encouragement in order to raise the overall standards of appraisal.[1]

Appraisal is a valuable process and the time and effort appraisees spend on their appraisal requires it to be done well. It has to be acknowledged that appraisals take a significant amount of time, time that could be spent looking after patients. Time spent on appraisal needs to be used efficiently and to good effect.

There is no place for poorly performed appraisals that are of little or no benefit to the appraisee. Indeed, badly performed appraisal is likely to lead to increased cynicism within the profession and further pressure on already busy doctors.

Badly performed appraisal is:

> no more than an exercise in gathering data and performing isolated analysis – a futile process at best.[2] (p.55)

Responsibility for the appraisal process working effectively lies with all those involved in its organisation and operation. One 'weak link' and the efforts and time spent by others can be undermined. This chapter looks primarily at the responsibilities of the appraiser, but also considers the important roles of those charged with administering appraisal and the vital role of the organisation in valuing and leading appraisal.

The NHS certainly has a way to go in considering the effectiveness of the organisation of appraisal. This is not a unique situation. Industry also falls into the trap of setting up expensive appraisal processes and then failing to ensure they are carried out well.[3,4]

This chapter considers a structure for quality assurance of appraisal, building on the reports of the National Association of Primary Care Educators[5] and, more recently, the National Clinical Governance Support Team.[6]

Quality assurance: an overview

If the aim of 'doing it well' is to be realised then the whole process needs to be considered. A clear understanding of the purpose of appraisal and the anchoring of appraisal in sound educational theory is important. Thorough preparations for appraisal, by appraiser and appraisee are vital. Well-chosen supporting information and correct use of the forms make this work more effectively. The selection, training and support of appraisers who have the ability to carry out a skilled appraisal interview are vital. All these will be to no avail if the appraiser and appraisee are not supported by an efficient administration.

Understanding the importance of appraisal leading on to relevant learning and professional development for the individual, as well as informing the development of the organisation, is also critical. Patient care is not likely to improve if appraisal sits as a stand-alone process unconnected with professional development and clinical governance structures.

The NCGST report[6] uses a checklist (Table 10.1) for the organisation to consider its success in developing a quality appraisal system. It is designed to be used as a simple self-assessment tool. It provides a useful summary of the topics to be considered and illustrates the need for the wide breadth of view in quality assurance.

Table 10.1 Quality assurance of appraisal: self-assessment checklist for organisations. Reproduced with permission from the National Clinical Governance Support Team[6]

	1	2	3
	Practice does not follow standards that should reasonably be expected	Practice in this area is sound, although progress can still be made	Practice in this area is excellent
The organisational ethos and commitment to appraisal			
The organisation has clearly identified resources to support appraisal	The allocation of resources is unclear and evaluations identify problems with resources supporting appraisal	There is a clear allocation of resources to support appraisal and this appears to be adequate	Evaluations demonstrate that the appraisal process is resourced well
An individual is responsible for leadership and development of the appraisal process	There is no defined leadership	An individual has the responsibility but does not have the time or resources to lead the appraisal process	The appraisal leadership is committed, informed and is able to lead the process effectively
An annual report is produced for the board	No annual report is produced	The annual report is incomplete or does not give clear information to the board	A well-produced annual report gives information to the board to allow individuals and the organisation to respond to appraisal
Appraisal is integrated with other processes for continuing professional development and clinical governance	It is not clear what place appraisal has in the organisational structure	Links exist between appraisal and CPD and governance but it is not clear how effective these links are	Appraisal is part of an integrated process for CPD and governance that is shown to work effectively
The organisation responds to needs identified in appraisal	It is unclear how the organisation responds to needs identified in appraisal	The trust has some processes to support individuals in addressing educational and/or developmental needs and also considers implications for the development of the trust.	There is a clear process to ensure that individuals are effectively supported in their development, barriers to development are addressed and the trust has clear planning and delivery of changes to address organisational developmental needs
Quality assurance	There is no clear process for quality assuring appraisal	The trust has processes to quality assure appraisal but these are not always effective	The trust has clear processes for monitoring the QA of appraisal and responds to needs identified

Table 10.1 (cont.)

	1	2	3
The confidentiality of the appraisal process is robust and trusted	It is unclear how effective any processes for confidentiality work	There is a clear policy that protects the confidentiality of the appraisal process	The confidentiality process is effective and, as evidence in evaluations, trusted by individuals
Actions to improve quality in these areas:			
Appraiser skills and training			
A defined person specification is used when selecting appraisers	There is no evidence that a clear person specification is used	A person specification exists and is used	A person specification is used, it is reviewed regularly and applied well
Appraisers are properly selected	It is not clear how appraisers are selected	Appraisers are selected at interview and a job description is available	There is a good selection procedure at interview, including lay representation, that enjoys the confidence of individuals in the organisation
Appointment as an appraiser depends on successful completion of training	Appraisers are not trained or it is unclear how they are trained	Appraisal training occurs	High-quality appraiser training is undertaken by all appraisers. This is provided by skilled trainers and feedback is given to appraisers on their strengths and weaknesses
There is a clear job description for appraisers	There is no job description	A job description exists	There is a job description that is regularly reviewed and accurately reflects the role of appraisers in the organisation
Appraisers are supported in their role	It is unclear what support, if any, exists for appraisers	Appraisers are supported by the appraisal lead and some links exist between appraisers	There is an appraisers group that meets regularly and offers support to appraisers and develops appraisers skills
Appraisers carry out an appropriate numbers of appraisals	It is unclear how many appraisals individual appraisers complete each year	There is a defined minimum and maximum number of appraisals completed by each appraiser annually	The number of appraisals completed by an appraiser complies with the trust's policy and reflects the needs of their own development

Table 10.1 (*cont.*)

	1	2	3
Assessment of appraisers skills	Appraisers skills are not assessed	Some assessment is made and feedback occurs to appraisers	Evaluation forms, the quality of Form 4s and observation of skills inform feedback to the appraiser. Reappointment as an appraiser depends on satisfactory performance and ongoing development of skills
Ongoing training of appraisers	It is unclear what further training appraisers undergo	Appraisers attend periodic retraining	Appraisers are actively involved in a developmental appraisers group, address needs identified in review of their performance and attend external training relevant to their needs on an annual basis. There is independent assessment of their skills on a 3-yearly basis
Actions to improve quality in these areas:			
The appraisal interview	1	2	3
The appraisal reviews the progress against the previous year's development plan	It is unclear how PDPs are reviewed	Appraisers review progress against development plans	Appraisers review progress against development plans as evidenced in Form 4s and in evaluations and this progress informs the subsequent year's development
The appraisal interview is challenging	It is unclear whether the interview is challenging	Appraisal appears to be appropriately challenging in most cases	Evaluation demonstrates that appraisers are able to challenge while remaining supportive to the appraiser
There is a clearly defined portfolio of evidence that informs appraisal	It is unclear how evidence is chosen to inform appraisal	An agreed evidence set is brought to appraisal	Defined and validated evidence informs both appraisal and revalidation and is useful for the appraiser and appraisee. This includes feedback from patients and 360-degree feedback from colleagues

Table 10.1 (*cont.*)

	1	2	3
There are clearly understood actions when the evidence informing appraisal in incomplete	It is unclear to appraisees and appraisers what should be done if information is incomplete	There is a written policy that outlines individuals' and the organisation's responsibilities if the evidence folder is incomplete	There is a written policy that is understood by all and mechanisms exist to support individuals in completing the evidence
The development plans are of a high standard and accurately reflect the appraisal interview	It is unclear whether the development plan reflects priorities identified in appraisal	The development plans appears to be well produced and considered	The development plans are excellent and evaluation shows they reflect individuals' needs
Appraisal takes place in an appropriate environment	There is no guidance on where appraisal takes place	There is guidance to ensure appraisal takes place in an appropriate environment	Guidance is effectively followed
Actions to improve quality in these areas:			
Systems and infrastructure supporting appraisal	1	2	3
There is sufficient administrative support for appraisal	There is no clearly identified administrative support and/or problems are identified in evaluations	There is dedicated administrative support that appears reasonably effective	Evaluations confirm the presence of effective administrative support for appraisal
Sufficient notice is given for appraisal	Insufficient time is available to prepare for appraisal	Sufficient time appears to be available	Sufficient time is available for appraiser and appraisee to prepare for appraisal and this is confirmed in evaluations of appraisal
Matching of appraiser and appraisee is well managed	It is unclear how matching occurs and/or problems are evident in the process	There is a process to match appraiser and appraisee	There is a clearly understood process to match appraiser and appraisee and a process exists for choice if a problem or conflict of interest is identified

Table 10.1 (*cont.*)

There is a complaints process should problems arise within the appraisal process	There does not appear to be a complaints process	A complaints process exists	A complaints process is produced, reviewed and is readily accessible to doctors in the organisation
Form 4s are signed by appraiser and appraisee	Forms 4s are not always signed	Form 4s are signed	Form 4s are legibly signed and GMC numbers appended to signatures
Form 4s are securely stored	Form 4s are not securely stored	Form 4s are securely stored	Form 4s are securely stored and there is evidence that access to them is robustly monitored
Doctors are appraised annually	It is unclear how many doctors are appraised or more than 5% of doctors are not appraised	At least 95% of doctors are appraised	At least 95% of doctors are appraised and an exception audit has taken place for doctors not appraised with actions to address any problems produced
Locums have been appraised	It is not known whether locums working in the organisation have been appraised	Locums working in the organisation have been appraised	Locums have been appraised and the date of their last appraisal recorded
Doctors working across organisations	The responsibility for carrying out appraisals is not clear	There is a policy to clarify where appraisal is done for doctors working within several organisations	There is a clear policy and a robust and confidential process for ensuring appraisal has occurred is in place that is understood by those doctors
The NHS Toolkit	The NHS Toolkit is not used	The NHS Toolkit is used	The NHS Toolkit is encouraged and arrangements for secure access understood

Actions to improve quality in these areas:

General comments and priorities identified

Name	Signature
Date	Position

By working through this checklist it can be seen that quality assurance need not be a complicated management tool. Instead, it can become part of a conscientious approach to everyday practice. The rest of this chapter focuses on some of the areas of quality assurance that are particularly applicable to the appraiser, the appraisal lead and the organisation.

The appraiser's role in quality assurance

The appraiser: right person for the right job

The appraiser needs to be the right person for the job. This is considered in more detail in Chapters 3 and 4 but a brief overview of the issues is repeated here.

Before they apply and are appointed, appraisers should think about why they want to be an appraiser. In secondary care, there has historically been little choice. Some doctors become appraisers by virtue of their position as medical director or clinical governance lead. In primary care, the first (and largest) tranche of appraisers were often given the positions without any formal appointment process.

More recently, person specifications for appraisers have been developed,[5–7] and examples of these are included in Chapter 11.

Table 10.2 combines some of the components of several appraiser person specifications and is included as a reminder of some of the key issues. While it is good to have consistency in selection, it is also important that there is room for local flexibility. This allows for the local needs of organisations to be met.

Table 10.2 Person specification for appraisers

Person specification for appraisers	Essential/ Desirable
Education	
Medical degree	E
Current GMC registration	E
Experience	
3 years since completion of specialist or GP training	E
Involvement in medical education	D
Skills and knowledge	
Good communication skills	E
Good interpersonal skills	E
Good organisational skills	E
Understanding of the purpose of medical appraisal	E
Understanding of equality and diversity best practice	E
Understanding of learning needs assessment	D
Knowledge of local networks for continuing professional development	D
Knowledge of resources to support individual learning	D
Personal qualities	
Self-motivated	E
Trustworthy and able to respect the confidentiality of the appraisal process	E
Enjoys respect of peers	E

The person specification should be able to discern well-motivated and skilled doctors who will make good appraisers. It is also essential that these appraisers enjoy the trust and respect of their colleagues.

The appraiser: initial training of medical appraisers

It is important to ensure that the right people put themselves forward and are selected for initial training. There also needs to be consistently good training for appraisers. Training should be able to equip, or at least start to equip, them with the skills needed to appraise. It is clear that not all appraisers have had good experiences of training and not all trained appraisers are good at their job.

It is currently the employing organisation's responsibility to commission appraisal training and to ensure that it is up to standard.[8] In some areas this responsibility is delegated to deaneries, or other bodies, who commission and monitor appraisal training on the employing organisation's behalf.

Appraisers have a real responsibility to ensure that they participate fully in the training and get the most out of it. Many training providers expect attendees to read or undertake other preparatory work before attending training and it is only fair that this is done. It is also important to complete the evaluation forms the training providers use. Such evaluations will (or certainly should) be used to constantly improve the training.

When embarking on a new area of interest or professional practice, it is sometimes difficult to admit that one has made a wrong decision. If the newly trained appraiser decides it is not, after all, 'for them', it is better to discuss this with the appraisal lead sooner rather than later.

The appraiser: ongoing training and support of medical appraisers

It is difficult to expect all appraisers to undergo their continuing professional development (CPD) as an appraiser in exactly the same way. Just as with clinical skills, individuals will differ in the areas they find most problematic. It is, however, vitally important to ensure that development occurs continually, and that the appraisers gain from this activity the support they need to enhance their appraisal skills.[6,8]

There are several models for such an appraiser support group and these are discussed more fully in Chapter 4. A regular forum to discuss ways of managing more challenging appraisals is often found to be useful. There also needs to be a system for appraisers to discuss difficulties quickly, should the need arise, with the appraisal lead or a more experienced appraiser.

In addition to this supportive function, there is the need to keep skills up to date and ensure that current thinking on appraisal is appreciated by appraisers.

The appraiser: reaccreditation of an appraiser's skills

There is no statutory requirement for appraisers to have their skills as an appraiser assessed on a regular basis. It is, of course, important that the appraiser role is covered in the appraiser's own NHS appraisal, probably under the section 'Teaching and training' or using an alternative appraisal model.

There are useful resources to encourage appraisers to think about their skills[7] and this book further explores this important area. It may be that, in time, organisations will require appraisers to be formally reaccredited on a regular basis. This has been piloted in a few areas in the UK.

This process should include:

- a review of the evaluations that have been made of the appraisers' appraisals
- a review of the skills they demonstrate at training days
- a review of the quality of the Form 4s and PDPs produced in appraisals
- a discussion about the progress in their development as appraisers.

While no definitive solution can be proposed at this stage, there needs to be consistency of standards across the UK. It is clear that appraisers need to keep their skills honed.

The appraiser: a contract

It is essential for an appraiser to have a contract with the organisation for which they are carrying out appraisals. While the legal responsibility for this lies with the employing organisation, there is sense in appraisers seeking a standard contract if there is not one in place. An example of a contract suitable for use in primary care is included in Chapter 12.

Professional bodies such as the British Medical Association (BMA) may be able to advise on the appropriateness of any contract. While it is to be hoped that appraisals will not be the subject of complaints and litigation (especially if done well), it is also important for the individual appraiser to satisfy themselves that they have adequate indemnity for their appraisal work. This needs to be clarified (preferably in writing) with the employer and also with the appraiser's medical indemnity organisation.

The appraiser needs to negotiate adequate time for the role with their employer. In secondary care, this will mean the appraiser has adequate protected time to ensure the job is done well. For independent contractors (such as GPs) this time will need to be paid for, either as a sessional payment or as an item of service fee under a service level agreement.

There is a need to ensure that time spent in preparing for appraisals, and the time the appraiser commits to training and continuing professional development as an appraiser, is properly resourced.

Those working in community and primary care settings will also want to see that travel and associated expenses are covered.

Doctors are often reticent to seek recognition of their additional work, but ensuring that the appraisal process is properly resourced is important to ensure its long-term development.

The appraisal lead's role in quality assurance

The responsibility

The appraisal process needs a leader. This should normally be a doctor. Many effective appraisal systems have medical leaders to take the process forward with highly competent managers to provide essential management and organisational leadership.

Leaders need to ensure that appraisers in their team are working effectively and conscientiously. They may run the local part of the appraiser group as well as ensuring that external training and support is appropriately commissioned to respond to the appraisers' needs.

Difficult appraisals will happen and there will always be issues that are not covered in guidance material and training. The appraisal lead should be available to assist and advise appraisers when these issues arise.

Leaders may well also take a responsibility in monitoring any changes in appraisal and ensuring that appraisers are kept up to date with these developments. Benchmarking local with national standards is an important part in the development of a robust process.

The appraisal lead: the annual report

There needs to be an annual report that accurately demonstrates the place of the appraisal process in the organisation. It should have a comprehensive remit to look at the areas outlined in Box 10.1.[9]

Box 10.1 The contents of a good annual appraisal report
- List individuals with responsibility for appraisal
- Activity levels (numbers of doctors appraised and (anonymised) reasons for any appraisals not done, e.g. maternity leave)
- Quality assurance of the appraisal process (internal processes, external processes, summary of evaluations and any research or developmental activity)
- Summary of individual learning needs
- Summary of individual developmental needs
- Organisational developmental needs
- Costs of the appraisal process
- Progress made by the organisation in addressing needs identified in previous year's appraisals

---

One of the most important parts of the appraisal report is to consider the progress against the previous year's report. Quality assurance should be an ongoing process that looks at the development of appraisal over time, rather than simply against a set of external criteria. Measuring achieves nothing unless the results are used to drive change and improvement.

Excellent examples of these reports exist and can be seen online at www. appraisalsupport.nhs.uk and can be downloaded free of charge. Reading somebody else's report can be encouraging in what can be a time-consuming, and sometimes difficult, job.

Within the appraisal report the appraisal lead needs to demonstrate that the information coming out of appraisal brings about change. The personal developmental needs arising out of appraisal should be summarised and collated by the

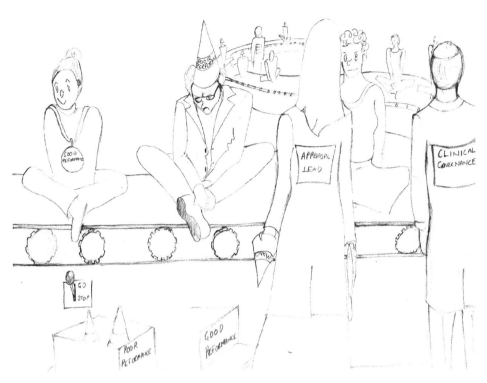

appraisal lead to produce a master list of needs for the individuals working within the organisation. This process needs to be understood by the appraisees and the appraisers in the organisation and there must be trust that the confidentiality of individuals' is absolute.

The collated learning needs should be shared with education and training committees within the Trusts (although clearly the structures of different organisations vary widely). This process should mirror structures for other health professionals.

Bespoke software can be used for this task. There is a strong case for such software to be further developed to encompass the needs of medical staff.

Collated learning needs should also be shared with tutors (clinical, college, primary care and GP tutors) working in trust and deanery settings. This informs the commissioning and provision of educational programmes.

There is little point in encouraging individuals to identify their needs if no opportunities are available to address those needs. This means that the forms used to collate the learning needs must communicate the needs in a way that can be used.

The report should also cover other developmental needs identified within the appraisal process.

The organisation's role in quality assurance

The success of appraisal lies in it being done well and in the appraisal being integrated into other processes for clinical governance and continuing professional development.

Appraisal is sometimes seen as a stand-alone activity, even as a replacement for continuing professional development. Clearly this is not the case. Appraisal is an activity that links other educational, clinical governance and quality improvement processes for the individual doctor and the organisation. It is an unfortunate reality that some have used the advent of appraisal as a convenient way of reducing the commitment to, and development of, programmes for continuing professional development.

The National Clinical Governance Support Team (NCGST) laid out four high-level indicators important in the quality assurance of medical appraisal (Box 10.2).[6] Every organisation should consider whether they embrace these indicators. These are the keystones of an effective appraisal process.

Box 10.2 The four pillars of quality assurance of appraisal

1 **Organisational ethos:** There is an unequivocal commitment from the highest levels of the host organisation to deliver a quality-assured system of appraisal that is fully integrated with other systems of quality improvement

2 **Appraiser selection, skills and training:** The host organisation has a process for selection of appraisers and appraiser skills are continually reviewed and developed

3 **Appraisal discussion:** The appraisal discussion is challenging and effective; it is informed by valid and verifiable supporting evidence

4 **Systems and infrastructure:** The supporting systems and infrastructure are effective and ensure that all doctors linked to the host organisation are supported and appraised annually

---

Putting these ideas into action requires effort, although great strides have been made in some parts of the UK, perhaps notably Scotland[10] and Wales.[11]

Good appraisers have good organisations behind them. The training and support that such organisations encourage in their appraisers is valuable. It is just as important for the success of appraisal that there is good administrative support and leadership. A well-organised appraisal system will lead to fewer frustrations and difficulties in such things as paperwork flow and the making of appraisal appointments. These are the nuts and bolts that are important to ensure the smooth running of the whole process.

Apart from the general picture painted by the high-level indicators above, how can this translate into practice?

The organisation: commitment

It is easy for a trust or other NHS organisation to pretend commitment and deliver little. All those in the NHS will recognise the difference between 'virtual' commitment (the evidence of which can be found in annual reports and mission statements but which does not exist on the ground) and 'real' commitment that values a system, invests in that system and develops the system.

This commitment needs individuals, supported from the very highest levels of the organisation, to work to develop appraisal. These key individuals must ensure that appraisers are working effectively, that the purpose of appraisal is understood and that the organisation responds to appraisal.

There are at least three levels in the organisation at which the response to appraisal needs to occur.

- **Individual learning needs:** ensuring that educational and developmental opportunities exist so that individuals can address their personal learning needs.
- **Individual developmental needs:** ensuring that the organisation responds to other developmental needs that have been identified in appraisal, such as difficulties in obtaining study leave, occupational health issues and other areas that may be alleviated by changing working practices.
- **Organisational developmental needs:** while the needs of individuals may provide the host organisation with lessons to be learned, there may be specific areas that arise out of appraisal that the trust needs to respond to as an important part of the risk management strategy. For example, problems with referrals to a particular department in the hospital that individuals find impedes their work should be addressed rather than avoided. It may also be that problems in other organisations (across the primary/secondary care divide for example) may appear. Patient care will be improved if these concerns are addressed.

The organisation: quality assurance

It seems to be navel gazing in the extreme to include quality assurance as a part of the quality assurance process. However, how quality assurance is organised is important.

The headings covered in this chapter need to be reviewed on a regular and ongoing basis, and the appraisal self-assessment checklist (Table 10.1) can be a tool to make this easier.

There needs also to be a system of external quality assurance to ensure that an objective view of the organisation and the appraisal process takes place. This may seem an expensive luxury but the appraisal process, as well as being important, is itself expensive, and the cost-effectiveness and use of valuable NHS resources needs to carefully considered.

There is great potential value in getting different individuals and organisations to carry out this quality assurance over time, bringing expertise and experience from different perspectives. Looking at an appraisal process from a medical education perspective might lead to different, but equally valid, recommendations.

The organisation: integration with other bodies and processes

Appraisal is not a stand-alone activity for individuals, replacing continuing professional development, nor is it a stand-alone process for the organisation, although many trusts in primary and secondary care appear to regard it as such.

The appraisal process needs to link with educational and clinical governance structures within the organisation and also at a local and regional level. Clearly this need not involve complicated paper chases or committee meetings. There should be an understanding that appraisal is important to all.

The organisation: confidentiality

The importance of confidentiality runs throughout this book and clearly many of the issues raised in appraisal are sensitive. There needs to be complete confidence, from appraisers and appraisees, in the confidentiality of the appraisal process.

The paperwork from appraisal (Form 4s and the PDP) should be stored securely. Only the named appraisal administrator and the named appraisal lead should have access to the forms (acting, in accordance with DoH guidance, on behalf of the chief executive[12,13]). The NHS Toolkit provides a similar level of security.

Appraisal paperwork should be sent securely within and without the organisation and clearly marked 'Appraisal in confidence' to ensure that it is not inadvertently opened.

The evaluation forms should include an item that asks appraisees to rate their confidence in the confidentiality of the appraisal process.

Conclusion

Quality assurance need not be a complicated or onerous task. It is the means to ensure that all the effort, innovation and resources being directed towards appraisal are effectively used to help doctors in their professional development. It provides the challenge to ensure that the appraisal process continues to improve. It enables the organisation to demonstrate that it is responding to the learning and developmental needs of doctors. This must, surely, lead to better patient care.

References

1 Dale B. *Managing Quality*. 4th ed. Oxford: Blackwell Publishing; 2003.
2 Jeska S. Evaluation: an important aspect of staff development service. *J Nurs Care Qual.* 1994. 8: 55–65.
3 Gillen T. *The Appraisal Discussion*. London: Chartered Institute of Personnel and Development; 1995.
4 Harvard B. *Performance Appraisals*. London: Kogan Page; 2001.
5 Lyons N. *Quality Assurance Standards for GP Appraisal*. Bury: National Association of Primary Care Educators; 2004.
6 National Clinical Governance Support Team. *Assuring the Quality of Medical Appraisal: report of the NHS Clinical Governance Support Team Expert Group*. Leicester: NCGST; 2005.
7 Chambers R *et al*. *The Good Appraisal Toolkit for Primary Care*. Oxford: Radcliffe Medical Press; 2004.
8 National Clinical Governance Support Team. *Defining the Evidence for Revalidation – Supporting the Royal College of General Practitioners. Collation of views from the NHS Clinical Governance Support Team Expert Group*. Leicester: NCGST; 2002.
9 Lyons N. How to write an annual appraisal report. In: Lyons N, editor. *ABC of Appraisal*. Bury: National Association of Primary Care Educators; 2004.
10 Murie J. GP appraisal recruitment in Scotland 2005. *BMJ Career Focus.* 2005; 331(7512): gp59–60.
11 GP Appraisal and CPD Unit. *GP Appraisal in Wales: annual report 2004/2005*. Cardiff: Cardiff University School of Postgraduate Medical and Dental Education; 2005.

12 Department of Health. *NHS Appraisal: appraisal for consultants working in the NHS*. London: DoH; 1999.
13 Department of Health. *NHS Appraisal: guidance on appraisal for general practitioners working in the NHS*. London: DoH; 2002.

Chapter 11

Developmental resources

This section of the book is designed to be a resource for appraisers and appraiser support groups to encourage development in appraisal skills. It is not designed to be read in one sitting, rather dipped into and used at appropriate times.

Appraisal skills development is an essential part of the delivery of high-quality appraisal. Many of the resources can be used as tools for personal reflection, but the most value is likely to be obtained if they are used in a group environment where different appraisers will bring their viewpoints to discussions.

It will cover the following topics.

- Ground rules for running small groups.
- Preparation form for appraisers.
- Giving feedback: the dos and the don'ts.
- Appraisal scenarios for individual reflection or group discussion.
- Using a simulated appraiser for practising appraisal discussion skills – small group session.
- Using a simulated appraiser for practising appraisal discussion skills – large group session.
- Further exercises for appraiser support group discussion.
- Reflective notes: a tool to reflect on difficult appraisals.
- Form 4 assessment tool.
- Personal development plan assessment tool.
- Appraiser training day: reflective notes.
- Appraiser training day: evaluation form.
- Websites and e-learning resources.

Ground rules for running small groups

It is necessary for a group that is discussing sensitive subjects, which may make individuals feel vulnerable, to feel secure and safe in the environment.[1,2] The group should ideally produce its own ground rules and thus feel able to 'own' the rules. However, it can be useful to have some rules up your sleeve if you are facilitating a session when the rules are being decided.

Checklist of rules that might be adopted by a group

Clear understanding of confidentiality
The group needs to agree and understand that the specifics of discussions must be completely confidential. However, the learning that comes out of the session is not. While this appears obvious, it goes wrong regularly and is worthy of careful thought.

Participation
Groups work better when all members participate.

Contribute when you have a contribution
There is a responsibility to contribute when you have an opinion or experience. However, we all recognise the person who makes a lot of noise without actually having much to contribute. . . .

Respect and honesty
Group members have a right to expect their viewpoint to be respected and for members to be honest in their statements. Honesty, however, does not need to be brutal or to cause hurt.

Listening and not 'rubbishing'
Some members will find it harder to participate than others. All should be listened to.

Preparation
If work requires some preparation, it is beholden that this is done. It is unfair to other members of the group to waste time in a meeting while one member reads the notes.

Timekeeping
Agreement is needed about starting and ending on time.

Interruptions
The group should decide what interruptions are allowable. Should mobiles be switched off or simply 'silenced'?

Time out
If emotional subjects are discussed the group may want to give itself the right to take a short break to ease tension.

Preparation form for appraisers

The appraiser may find it useful (as discussed in Chapter 6) to have a structured format for recording notes during the appraisal discussion. This example, looking at good clinical care, has been taken from a complete document which includes a similar page for each of the headings of *Good Medical Practice*.[3]

The whole document is available on the NAPCE website.

Appraiser's preparation form
Good clinical care
Examples of good practice

Areas to explore

Notes during the discussion

Notes during reflection

Giving feedback: the dos and don'ts

The dos . . .

Give it with care	To be useful, feedback requires the giver to want to help, not hurt, the other person
Let the recipient invite it	Feedback is most effective when the receiver has invited the comments. Doing so indicates that the receiver is ready to hear the feedback and give that person an opportunity to specify areas of interest/concern
Encourage self-criticism	People are willing to accept criticism when they have recognised their own strengths and weaknesses. Start by encouraging them to appraise themselves and then build on their own insights

Be specific	Good feedback deals with particular incidents and behaviour. Making vague or woolly statements is of little value. The most helpful feedback is concrete and covers the area of interest specified by the receiver
Outline the positive	By making feedback constructive you will be helping the receiver to find out what needs to be done rather than just telling them what they are doing wrong. Always look for areas of improvement rather than what went wrong
Avoid evaluative judgements	The most useful feedback describes behaviours without value; labels such as 'irresponsible', 'unprofessional', or even 'good' or 'bad' are unhelpful. If the recipient asks you for a judgement, be sure to state that this is your opinion
Make the feedback actionable	To be most useful, feedback should concern behaviour that can be changed by the receiver. Feedback concerning matters outside the control of the receiver is less useful and often causes resentment
Balance the positive and negative	Always begin and end with a positive for each point you are making. Avoid giving all the positive points at the beginning or end of the whole feedback session. This allows the receiver to hear a more balanced view
Balance the timing of positives and negatives	Positive feedback on its own allows no room for improvement and negative feedback alone is discouraging
Choose the right time and place	The most useful feedback is given at a time and place that make it easy for the receiver to hear it, e.g. away from other people and distractions. It should be given sufficiently close to the particular event being discussed for it to be fresh in mind. Enough time should be allocated to explore any issues raised

. . . and the don'ts

Deny the other persons feelings	You need to demonstrate empathy with the other person's feelings and experience. Otherwise they will not feel valued. The other person may spend time thinking of defensive responses rather than listening to your suggestions
Be vague	If you are vague the other person cannot be clear about what you are suggesting should be changed and how
Take for granted the person has understood	Ask the other person to summarise what you have said to ensure that you have expressed yourself clearly and to avoid misunderstandings
Bring in third parties	You are the person giving the feedback. You should let third parties give their own feedback. If you have to rely on a third party or hearsay, you need to consider why you are giving the feedback
Be negative	Giving feedback is not always a comfortable experience. However, even if there is something important that needs to be addressed, the 'how' of telling needs to have a positive spin of what can be improved rather than what was wrong
Be destructive	It is easy to be unintentionally destructive and this needs to be avoided at all costs. It can destroy the relationship between the giver and receiver of the feedback irreparably

Be judgemental	It is important for the person giving feedback to remember that there is usually more than one way to achieve a result. Saying an action was 'good' is judgemental, while saying it was 'effective' gives more useful feedback
Bring up behaviours that the person cannot help	Stammers, tics and other repetitive habits are inherent and cannot be changed, or at least need input that is beyond the remit of an appraiser training session
Be overly impressed	Being overly impressed can sound patronising. It could also bring some resentment into the group
Be aggressive	There is no place for aggressiveness in giving feedback, it is destructive in any situation. Even if the receiver is aggressive, the person giving feedback must not respond in kind. They need to challenge the receiver's behaviour and try to get to a place where a reasonable dialogue can resume.

Appraisal scenarios for individual reflection or group discussion

A series of scenarios are presented that can be used for reflection or to stimulate discussion. They can be readily adapted for role play. If used in a group, the session organiser needs to consider why the scenario is being used and what learning points the group might be looking for.

Scenarios can be used to help relatively inexperienced appraisers consider more complex situations or to explore significant events that have happened in real life without compromising the confidentiality of the actual situation.

Questions that individuals can be asked include the following:

- What issues does this situation raise?
- How would you approach this appraisee?
- What are your alternative approaches to the problem?
- Would you stop the appraisal in this situation? If so, on what grounds?
- Who might you discuss this situation with?
- How would you document the situation?

The choice of questions for the small group to use and the choice of scenario may depend on the objectives of the training session.

Doctor A has clearly prepared well for appraisal and presents a comprehensive development plan with action points prepared under each of the appraisal headings, each justified and evidenced. He has over 30 action points but feels that as he is well organised and motivated this quantity is appropriate.

During the appraisal he appears reluctant to discuss how he came to choose the action points . . . they seem reasonable ideas but don't seem to particularly related to Doctor A, in fact you wonder if you have seen the list before somewhere, perhaps even in one of the free medical newspapers.

Doctor B is a well-respected member of the medical community, indeed you feel some trepidation that you are being asked to appraise her. However, it very rapidly becomes apparent that she has many problems, and you are concerned that her involvement in medical committee work appears to have increased since the breakdown of her marriage. When you explore this with her, she appears very distressed and will not discuss her feelings . . .

Doctor C is a wise and respected consultant. The appraisal goes well, and you complete your Form 4 with record speed. Just as you are leaving Doctor C asks who will be appraising Doctor D . . . as he is concerned that Doctor D has a significant alcohol problem that other colleagues are attempting to cover up . . .

Doctor E appears very friendly and helpful during the appraisal. You become concerned that he seems to be expecting you to negotiate a PDP that is, to be charitable, light in content. He is expecting you to support him in this as the pressure of trust work is becoming too much and, clearly, there is not sufficient time to tackle everything . . . is there?

Doctor G thanks you for an excellent, challenging appraisal. You have really helped her look at her development goals and she is keen to have an appraisal with you next year, so you can further discuss the ideas she is developing in her practice. It was such a pity that the appraisal she had last year had been such a waste of time, as that appraiser seemed more concerned with his own development than hers . . .

Doctor H is doing OK. You have no concerns about his fitness to perform his duties but he appears unwell and perhaps depressed. He is registered with a close colleague with whom he went to medical school and you can see samples of antidepressants clearly visible in his office.

Doctor I is a part-time sessional doctor who has worked for many years as a missionary abroad. He has three letters of praise, which appear to be from friends. He has had an informal complaint, which he says has been sorted (although no details are available). He brings a video to the appraisal and asks to show it to demonstrate his consultation skills. You agree to watch it but see abrupt conversations, no eye contact, closed questioning and a very judge-mental style of practice.

Doctor J is worried. She is, as far as you can tell, a hard-working and conscientious doctor. She has never been involved in audit and confesses she does not really understand the principles of audit. She does not want to start now, but realises that it is an expectation she should fulfil. She wants advice about what to do.

Doctor K is very distracted from practice as his mother is ill and his father is very frail and dependent. Concentration in the outpatients department is difficult and his secretary is always interrupting with questions from the family, social services and the hospital where his mother is.

Doctor L is enthusiastic about appraisal (indeed enthusiastic about every-thing) and has many interests and ideas. The appraisal paperwork is sparse and the positive ideas are not backed up by any evidence, paperwork or substance . . .

Doctor M is a respected doctor who works hard. His marriage is on the rocks and he feels he cannot discuss it with anybody. He is finding it hard to work and is not getting much sleep. He wants to discuss his choices and career development with his appraiser now that he has met a potential new partner, and feels that discussing anything else is pointless when his mental energies are consumed by his predicament.

Exercises and resources for appraisal leads

Using simulated appraisees (professional role players) for practising appraisal discussion skills: small group

This session plan is based on an appraiser support group working with a simulated appraisee.

Any of the resource scenarios in this chapter can be adapted to be used with simulated appraisees. This session is useful for both new and experienced apprai-sers to improve their communication skills.

The role player

Role players may or may not be actors. There is a significant difference between an actor and a role player. Generally, an actor will act to a script, and some are very good at improvising. Role players on the other hand respond to the appraiser and react to the way the appraiser behaves (e.g. a closed question will get a mono-syllabic answer, while an open question will reveal more information).

Attention should be paid to the choice of role player from the pool available. A few have worked as simulated patients and understand NHS jargon. Others have been specifically trained to play doctor roles, such as appraisees or doctors in difficulty. It is useful to have a role player who is quick at understanding the basic principles when a scenario is being developed 'on the hoof'.

The scenario

The role player needs to be given time to prepare the scenario in advance. The headings are important, and the content should not be too complicated. Special attention needs to be paid to the learning outcomes and the specific skills the appraisers wish to practise.

Setting the scene

- Establish initial rapport:
    - welcome, introductions
    - explore and discuss how this session fits in with appraisers' overall learning
    - outline the timing of the session, explain the aims and methods of the session, particularly a structure for giving feedback
    - demonstrate interest and concern.
- Develop a shared agenda for the group:
    - appraisers' issues
    - appraisee's issues
    - appraisal lead or trainer's (facilitator's) issues.
- Explain that this is a chance to practise important areas before doing so in real life. It is not a judgemental exercise but an opportunity to practise and rehearse in safety, as many times as they need, some of the skills that might be helpful to them.
- Describe the specific scenario to be used as a basis for the learning in enough detail to orientate the group.
- Ask the group to discuss the general issues that the scenario provides. Start by identifying the appraiser's initial agenda.
- Encourage one of the appraisers to start the process, pointing out that each person in turn will give raw material to work on when they undertake the discussion:
    - what would you like to practice and refine and get feedback on?
    - what are your personal objectives for the discussion? put on flipchart/board
    - how can the group help you best?
    - what would you like feedback on? Is there anything in particular you want us to watch for?

Prepare the whole group to watch the discussion

- Set up the room and make sure all are ready and roles worked out.
- Is there anything else the appraiser would like to know about the scenario to make it real, and make it work?
- Emphasise to the appraiser that it is OK to stop and start and break for help whenever they like.

- Suggest how long the discussion might go on for, or whether the facilitator should stop proceedings at an appropriate time. (It is difficult balancing the individual appraiser's needs with the need for 'everyone to have a go'.)
- Instruct the group to write down specific words and actions as an aid to descriptive feedback.
- One of the group can be set the task of identifying specific areas to feed back.
- Record the content of the appraisal discussion rather than the process.

Watch the appraisal discussion

- Allow the group several moments to collect their thoughts.
- Identify the one or two most important points they would like to bring up in feedback, making sure to provide a balance between what worked and what caused problems.
- It is the facilitator's responsibility to consider where to place feedback on what worked well.

Acknowledge the appraiser's feelings

- How do you feel? How did that go?

Refine the individual's agenda and identify the desired outcomes

- Can we go back to your agenda on the flipchart before the role play? Has it changed? Did new areas of difficulty crop up? Can we identify the problems?
- What would you like to have achieved differently? Given the problems we have identified what different outcomes would you like to explore?
- Facilitator to listen, clarify, summarise, check.

Feedback and re-rehearsal (whole group)

- Negotiate with the appraiser the best way to feed back on the appraisal discussion – choose which area to focus on.
- Start with the appraiser. Options here include:
  - Have you already got some thoughts about how you might approach this differently now that you are clear about the outcome you'd like to get to?
  - You obviously have a clear idea of what you would like to try next . . .
  - You've defined the problem and made a suggestion . . . would you like to have another go?
  - What went well/less well in relation to your specific objectives?
- Be explicit about the outcome for specific areas under discussion:
  - What are you and the appraisee trying to achieve? What were you getting at with that question?
- Get descriptive feedback from the group.
- When participants make suggestions, ask the appraiser if they would like to try this out or if they would like another group member to have a go.
- Invite the role player to add their insights.
- Rerun the scenario from a point where an alternative approach has been identified.
- Elicit thoughts and feelings of appraiser and role player, including the outcomes they wanted to achieve at various points in the appraisal discussion.

- Remember to:
  - practise and re-rehearse new techniques after suggestions from the group
  - make sure to balance positive and negative feedback
  - utilise role player feedback
  - demonstrate the skills yourself when appropriate
  - use the adapted Calgary–Cambridge guide.

Skills spotting, tape review

- Look at the micro-skills of communication and the exact words used.
- Use the careful notes of precise content made by the observers or video replay.

Introduce facilitator's agenda/teaching points: generalising away

- Add in facilitator's ideas and thoughts.
- Appropriately introduce theory, research and wider discussion.

Closing the session

- Clarify with appraiser that the agenda has been covered.
- Be very careful to balance what worked well and what didn't by the end.
- Ask what everyone has learned and whether the feedback was useful and felt acceptable.
- Summarise by pulling together learning points and reflection.
- Check that evaluations and reflective notes will be completed.

Using a simulated appraisee for practising appraisal discussion skills: issues for large groups

Big groups are not safe environments to allow individuals to try out new skills in public as the trust and confidentiality required cannot easily be developed. However, a 'demonstrator appraiser' can role play a scene with the simulated appraisee if it is carefully scripted.

Group discussion

The scenario is thrown open to the participants to discuss in groups the issues that the scenario raises, and their thoughts are then put on a flipchart.

Role play continues with a pre-planned solution

The participants will no doubt have a view and some will disagree with the 'demonstrator appraiser's' action. If time allows, another suggested way of handling the situation may be tried.

This method is a way of bringing the scenario to life and encouraging appraiser support groups to consider using a role player in their training sessions.

Further exercises for appraiser support group discussion (could be adapted for individual reflection)

Three further examples of exercises that may be useful for those who lead appraiser support groups are given below.

Small group work exercise 1: Limits of the appraiser role

Exercise length: 45 minutes

Subdivide the appraiser group into small groups of four or five appraisers and set them the following task. They should discuss under what circumstances the appraisal should be stopped in the event of the following issues presenting during the appraisal discussion:

- drug or alcohol abuse
- mental or physical illness
- self-prescription of drugs
- inappropriate behaviour with a patient
- not engaging in the appraisal process
- disclosure of evidence suggesting poor performance in the appraisee
- disclosure by the appraisee of serious poor performance in a colleague.

- Under what circumstances would you expect to stop the appraisal?
- How would you stop the appraisal process?
- What would you do next?
- What are your responsibilities in this situation?

Small group work exercise 2: The Form 4

Exercise length: 30 minutes

Subdivide the appraiser group into small groups of four or five appraisers and set them the following tasks.

- What is the purpose of the Form 4?
- Considering each purpose, for whom is the form written?
- How can you ensure the form is 'fit for purpose'?

Small group work exercise 3: The difficult appraisal

Exercise length: 45 minutes

Subdivide the appraiser group into small groups of three appraisers and set them the following task. They should take five minutes to prepare individually and then spend five minutes in turn describing their appraisal. When all have 'presented' their appraisal they should work as a group on the general questions.

- Think of the most difficult appraisal that you have done and describe the setting in a few sentences.
- What were the issues or concerns that made it difficult?
- Describe the strategies that you were able to successfully use and consider why they worked. Did others not work so well, and if not do you know why?
- What was the outcome?

Then as a group consider the following.

- What common themes have you discussed?
- How might you better prepare for such eventualities in the future?

Tool to reflect on difficult appraisals

All doctors should be recording evidence of their reflection. It is useful for appraisers to practise this skill in their own development as appraisers. The pro forma below offers a simple tool to capture the thinking around a difficult appraisal. It can be kept in the portfolio of evidence of reflective practice.

A difficult appraisal: reflective notes

Name: Date:

Think of the most difficult appraisal that you have done, and describe the setting in a few sentences.

What were the issues or concerns that made it difficult?

What did you do?

What worked well?

What did not work well?

What was the outcome of the appraisal?

What could you try in a similar situation?

Form 4 assessment tool

This simple assessment tool to help consider the quality of a Form 4 is adapted from the work of Di Jelley[4] and Amar Rughani.[5]

Legible	It may be more difficult to organise, but typed rather than handwritten documents tend to be better. Web-based systems such as the Welsh or the NHS Appraisal Toolkit achieve this naturally
Accurate in detail	Each statement should be honest and justifiable. The Form 4 is not the arena to introduce new topics or ideas!
Accurate in overview	The overall sense of the document should accurately represent the discussion. There should not be omissions or emphases that alter the overall sense and value of the discussion
Concise	It is not an academic essay. The comments should be succinct
Specific	The use of vague statements is not helpful
Positive	Strengths, successes and achievements should be included, not simply areas for development
Dynamic	The form should refer to the development planned in the previous year's appraisal, summarise the current year and look forward to the next
Objective and evidenced	This is not the place for speculation or reflection. All statements should be justifiable and objective. 'Softer' statements should only be included if the sense and purpose is clear
Free of bias and prejudice	The objectivity goes further as the appraiser should ensure that any prior knowledge of the appraisee or their role does not influence the document
Fit for purpose	The sum of the points in the Form 4 should be able to fulfil all the purposes listed above
Acceptable to the appraisee	Above all else the appraiser should ensure that they have not led the appraisee into accepting a document that is not acceptable or fair to them.

Personal development plan assessment tool

This series of questions to use when considering the PDP is derived from many different sources, pulled together by Dr Robin Gleek and the team at Cheshire West PCT and reproduced here with his kind permission.

As part of the development of the appraisal scheme, we have redesigned the PDP template for 2005 (CWPCT).

The appraiser will consider the following questions when completing and signing off the PDP.

1   Was the learning carried out in any planned way? As part of a PDP for the year, towards identified needs, as part of a programme or extended course leading to a qualification?

2 Were the learning methods used appropriate? For the learning needs, for the GP's learning style, for what was available and accessible to them.

3 Has the GP reflected on the learning? E.g. have the main learning points from a course been identified, has a personal learning record been kept?

4 Has the learning been successful, and made a difference? Has the GP applied it and changed the way they do things, e.g. has the learning been shared with colleagues or resulted in a new practice protocol?

5 Does the evidence of learning match the original learning need? E.g. clinical audit demonstrates a change in practice?

6 Has the GP carried out a personal review of the last year's education and learning? Things that went well, things that went less well, as part of Form 3 or separately?

7 Have outstanding or new learning needs been identified for the year ahead? Identified in a learning record, in Form 3 or incorporated into a draft PDP for the coming year?

The important areas to cover are:

- action to maintain skills and the level of service to patients
- action to develop or acquire new skills
- action to change or improve existing practice.

Appraiser training day: reflective notes

Every educational event should result in reflection by the participants. This should be recorded in a simple format and kept for their portfolio. An example of a form to record reflection is shown below.

Appraiser training day: reflective notes

Date of training:

Venue:

Action points from the training are:

I will know I have put these action points into action when I have . . .

Any other comments ?

Please include this form in your personal learning portfolio

Appraiser training day: evaluation

Similarly, every educational event should be evaluated. An example of an evaluation form is included below.

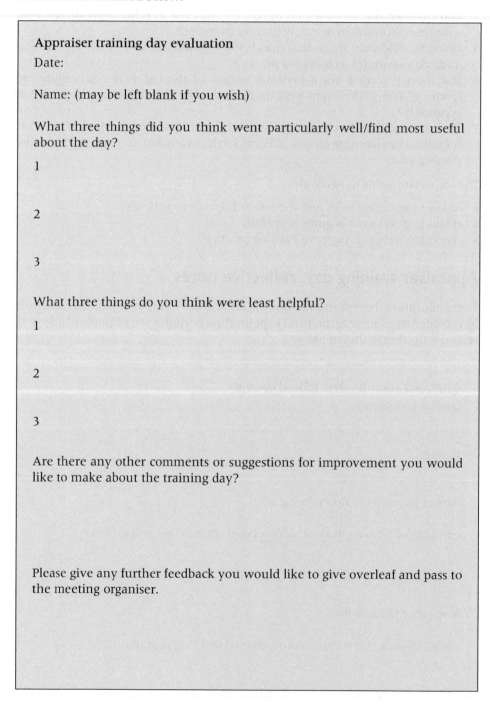

Appraiser training day evaluation

Date:

Name: (may be left blank if you wish)

What three things did you think went particularly well/find most useful about the day?

1

2

3

What three things do you think were least helpful?

1

2

3

Are there any other comments or suggestions for improvement you would like to make about the training day?

Please give any further feedback you would like to give overleaf and pass to the meeting organiser.

Websites and e-learning resources

Websites change and links are difficult to keep up to date, and sometimes move or become defunct. Often if you are hunting for a resource, one of the search engines will provide you with a selection of suitable sites with relevant information. Here are a few sites of particular relevance to appraisers.

Sites that support appraisers or provide information on appraisal

www.appraisalsupport.nhs.uk
This NHS site run by the National Clinical Governance support team aims to support high-quality appraisals. Resources are available for (free) download and a discussion forum is available for appraisers facing particular issues.

www.appraisals.nhs.uk
A secure password-protected site that provides access to the electronic toolkit for appraisals. A key benefit is the provision of a summary statement, including a personal development plan, generated automatically based on the information entered.

www.napce.net
This is site of the National Association of Primary Care Educators and provides resources to support educators and appraisers working in primary care (some resources only available to members).

http://primarycare-wales.org.uk/appraisal/process.php
www.nes.scot.nhs.uk/GP_Appraisal/
The Welsh and the Scottish primary care appraisal processes lay out excellent examples of good practice and are worth exploring for all appraisers.

www.shef.ac.uk/scharr
Sheffield University School of Health and Related Research (ScHARR) has published a report on GP appraisal and includes guidance on best practice.

www.shef.ac.uk/scharr/hpm/extendingappraisals.pdf
Guidance on appraisals for sessional GPs.

www.appraisal-skills.com
An educational interactive package for developing appraisal skills.

www.BAMM.co.uk
The British Association of Medical Managers website links to the standard documentation for appraisal. Also details of training on appraisals.

www.gmc-uk.org
The GMC website has information on *Good Medical Practice* and continuing professional development.

www.nasgp.org.uk
Information on appraisals for sessional GPs.

Sites that provide resources that appraisers might want to 'signpost'

www.bmjlearning.com
This site provides excellent learning resources and self-assessment tools.

www.doctors.net.uk
This site gives useful educational material as well as other information of relevance to doctors in their professional lives.

www.onmedica.net
This site gives useful interactive tutorials and self-assessment resources and records the activity in a log for the user.

www.rcplive.ac/
This online learning resource provides an imaginative approach to learning and is accessible to members of other Colleges as well as the RCP.

www.gpnotebook.co.uk
A useful source of medical information in the form of an easy to use medical encyclopaedia.

www.gplearning.co.uk
Desktop portfolio for recording personal learning.

www.doctoronline.nhs.uk
Information on education, clinical guidelines, etc.

www.easterngp.co.uk/pages/co/gpcpdretainer_all.php
Retained doctor support and advice.

www.bma.org.uk/ap.nsf/Content/refugeedrinitiative2006?OpenDocument& Highlight=2,refugee
Useful insights into the problems facing refugee doctors.

www.bmjcareers.com
The *British Medical Journal*'s career section contains useful articles on appraisal.

www.cybermedicalcollege.com
Information on appraisal and CPD for healthcare professionals. Backed by the Royal College of Physicians and Surgeons of Glasgow and the Royal College of Anaesthetists.

www.pdptoolkit.co.uk
Eastern Deanery Postgraduate GP education site with information on appraisals and PDPs.

www.the-mdu.com/gp/services/risk_management/assess1/index.asp
Risk assessment tools for revalidation; covers four of the headings in *Good Medical Practice*, including good communication, record keeping and handling complaints.

www.emispdp.com
EMIS education and PDP site.

www.problembasedlearning.com
Resources for problem-based learning.

www.modern.nhs.uk/protocolbasedcare
A step-by-step guide to developing protocols.

www.nelh.nhs.uk
National Electronic Library for Health provides access to Cochrane Library, Clinical Evidence, *BNF*, etc.

www.jr2.ox.ac.uk/bandolier
Evidence-based medicine.

www.nice.org.uk
Reviews, technology assessments and appraisals.

www.natpact.nhs.uk
Website for sharing information on developments in primary care, includes useful tools, discussion forums, etc.

www.themindgym.com
Tips and techniques on a variety of topics such as conflict resolution, stress management, time management, etc.

Supporting doctors

Contact details for organisations offering support to doctors

National Counselling Service for Sick Doctors	0870 241 0535 www.ncssd.org.uk An independent organisation providing a confidential advice and information service for doctors whose state of health may be compromising their ability to treat patients safely
British Doctors and Dentists Group	020 7487 4445 Doctors recovering from chemical dependency, monthly group meetings
Doctors Support Network	0870 321 0642 Friendly, relaxed network for doctors who have or have had mental health problems

Samaritans	08457 90 90 90
Doctors' Support Line	0870 765 0001 www.doctorssupportline.org Staffed by trained volunteer doctors. Confidential and anonymous service to talk about work and personal concerns
The Cameron Fund London WC1H 9BR	Help specifically for GPs and their dependants when they are in difficulties
Society for the Relief of Widows and Orphans of Medical Men London	A friendly society to look after its members and their dependants, but occasionally offers help to other doctors and their dependants
GP Care	Free phone 0800 214 307 24 hours, 365 days
BMA counselling (BMA members only)	08459 9200 169 24-hour support with immediate access to trained counsellors

Fitness to work

- Cox RAF, Edwards FC, Palmer K, editors. *Fitness for Work: the medical aspects*. 3rd ed. Oxford: Oxford University Press/Faculty of Occupational Medicine; 2000.
- Disability Discriminations Act 1995. www.disability.gov.uk
- Dawson A, Tylee A, editors. *Depression: social and economic time bomb*. London: BMJ Books (on behalf of the World Health Organization); 2001.

References

1 Tiberius R. *Small Group Teaching: a trouble shooting guide*. London: Kogan Page; 1999.
2 Jacques D. *Learning in Groups*. 3rd ed. London: Kogan Page; 2000.
3 General Medical Council. *Good Medical Practice*. 3rd ed. London: GMC; 2001.
4 Jelley D. *Writing a Good Form 4 – why bother?* Newcastle: Northern Deanery; 2005.
5 Rughani A. *GP Appraisal Forms 3 and 4: providing guidance and setting standards*. Sheffield: South Yorkshire and South Humber Deanery; 2003.

Chapter 12

Administrative resources

This chapter gives examples of material that has been developed to support the delivery of high quality appraisal systems.

One of the driving forces for development of appraisal has been the enthusiasm and drive of so many individuals across the UK in implementing a successful appraisal process. The diversity that has resulted has inevitably led to some significant inconsistencies.

This chapter includes examples of material that has been used to support the appraisal process. These will need careful adaptation before being used by any other organisation and updated to reflect current practice. They do, however, serve to illustrate issues raised in this book.

- Person specification for appraiser.
- Specimen job description for appraiser.
- Specimen primary care trust appraiser contract.
- Specimen evaluation form (for appraisee to complete).
- Specimen evaluation form (for appraiser to complete).
- Specimen example of health sign-off statement.

The latest examples of forms and resources may also be viewed at the National Clinical Governance Support Team appraisal site www.appraisal.support.nhs.uk

Person specification for appointment of a medical appraiser

Example 1. Adapted from the National Clinical Governance Support Team Report Assuring the Quality of Medical Appraisal[1]

Person specification for medical appraiser	Essential/Desirable
Education	
Medical degree	E
GMC registration	E
Completion of appraisal training before appointment	E
Experience	
3 years since completion of specialist or GP training	E
Involvement in medical education or training	D

Person specification for medical appraiser	*Essential/Desirable*
Skills, aptitudes and knowledge	
Interpersonal and communication skills	E
Understanding of the appraisal process	E
Understanding of equality and diversity best practice	E
Understanding of needs assessment	D
Knowledge of local professional development and education structures	D
Personal qualities	
Motivated and conscientious	E
Enjoying respect of colleagues	E
Health and physical abilities	
Psychologically capable of work as an appraiser	E

Example 2. Central Cheshire Primary Care Trust

Knowledge skills and attributes	*Essential*	*Desirable*
General practitioner GP working currently, or within the past two years, as a GP principal	√	
Have been a GP in practice (i.e. on a health authority list or supplementary list) for a minimum of five years	√	
Not be employed directly by a PCT as a clinical governance lead or executive committee chair	√	
Undertakes training or development of staff or GP tutor, trainer type role		√
Prepared to express and develop an interest in GP education and facilitation skills	√	
Effective interpersonal skills (ability to build up good rapport with participants)	√	
Evidence of good listening skills and patience to assist with difficulties	√	
Ability to demonstrate open, non-judgemental attitude and accept challenges to existing ideas	√	
Proven record for trustworthiness among colleagues	√	
Ability to be flexible	√	
Able to demonstrate commitment and give sufficient time to performing the appraiser role	√	

Specimen job description for a medical appraiser

Example 1. Adapted from the Essex Scheme[2]

Role:	GP appraiser
Accountable to:	PCO clinical governance lead or director of public health
Responsible to:	PCO clinical governance lead

Job summary
To appraise general practitioners in a supportive and developmental manner, to improve GP morale and clinical care.

Appraisal is a professional process of constructive dialogue, designed to give GPs feedback on past performance, chart continuing progress and identify development needs. It is seen as a formative and developmental process carried out by a GP who has been trained in carrying out appraisal.

Key tasks and responsibilities
To carry out a minimum of two, and a recommended maximum of 25, appraisals each year based on the GMC's core headings set out in the *Good Medical Practice* document.

To arrange to undertake GP appraisals at the convenience of the appraisee, in a comfortable setting, free from interruptions and distractions. The discussion should be based on accurate, relevant and up-to-date information and seek to identify:

- achievements and challenges in the past 12 months (clinical and non-clinical), seen where relevant in the context of earlier appraisals
- service, practice and (where relevant) wider objectives for the next year and beyond
- personal (and if appropriate to a discussion about the individual, the practice's) development needs and how these needs can be met.

To complete all standardised documentation in sequence to provide a formal, supportive, consistent structure to the appraisal process. Key points and outcomes of the discussion must be fully documented and copies held by the appraisee. An agreed and signed copy of the appraisal summary document (Form 4) must be forwarded, in confidence, to:

- the clinical governance lead at the PCO (for contracted GPs)
- the sessional GP team (where agreed by appraisee for sessional GPs).

To conclude the appraisal discussion by assisting the appraisee to set down, as an action plan, the agreements which have been reached and provide ongoing support for reviewing and updating personal development plans.
At the request of the appraisee, agree a date to undertake an appraisal review,

six months following each appraisal, to discuss progress towards achievement of personal development plans and provide further assistance.
To identify any areas where separate peer review by colleagues with relevant
expertise and knowledge is required and agree the necessary arrangement,
taking account of any such feedback in the appraisal summary.

To undertake two days' approved appraisal training, attend regular
appraisal support meetings and be prepared to be appraised as an appraiser.
Professional support to be provided by appraisal support group.

To recognise potentially serious performance issues where a colleague's
health, conduct or performance poses a threat to patients. It would be
exceptional for such serious concerns to be first identified at appraisal, but
both appraisers and appraisees need to recognise that as registered medical
practitioners, patients must be protected.

To comply with the requirements of the Data Protection Act in respect to
the storing and use of all documentation and to undertake to return to the
PCO clinical governance lead any outstanding documentation should your
role as appraiser cease.

Specimen primary care trust appraiser contract

Example 1. Adapted from Central Cheshire Primary Care Trust

STATEMENT OF TERMS AND CONDITIONS OF ENGAGEMENT

HONORARY CONTRACT

The main purpose of GP appraisal is to appraise general practitioners in a
supportive and developmental manner to improve morale and clinical care.
Appraisal for GPs is a professional process of constructive dialogue, designed
to give GPs feedback on past performance, chart continuing progress and
identify development needs. It is seen as a formative and developmental
process carried out by a GP who has been trained in carrying out appraisal.
Central Cheshire Primary Care Trust (CCPCT) expects all its employees to
support and enhance its care and overall quality of service. It also expects
each of its staff to act in a way to justify public confidence and enhance the
good reputation of Central Cheshire PCT.

PERSONAL
Name:
Address:

Appointment: GP appraiser
Service or Area: Primary care development

Date of appointment: September 2002
Review date (one year from appointment): September 2003

Compensation payments: £400 per completed appraisal plus two sessions of locum reimbursement at the CCPCT rate

SERVICES TO BE PROVIDED BY THE APPRAISER

So long as s/he shall continue to serve the PCT under the terms of this Agreement, the GP appraiser will undertake the appraisal programme outlined below.

To carry out up to 12 GP appraisals each year based on the GMC's core headings set out in the *Good Medical Practice* document. To give up to two months' notice in advance of the date of each appraisal and completing all preparatory information gathering and documentation for discussion at least two weeks before the appraisal date.

To arrange to undertake GP appraisals at the convenience of the appraisee, in a comfortable setting, free from interruptions and distractions. The discussion should be based on accurate, relevant and up-to-date information and seek to identify:

- achievements and challenges in the past 12 months (clinical and non-clinical), seen where relevant in the context of earlier appraisals
- service, practice and (where relevant) wider objectives for the next year and beyond
- personal (and if appropriate to a discussion about the individual, the practice's) development needs and how these needs can be met.

To complete all standardised documentation in sequence to provide a formal, supportive, consistent structure to the appraisal process. Key points and outcomes of the discussion must be fully documented and copies held by the appraiser and appraisee. An agreed and signed copy of the appraisal summary document (Form 4) must be forwarded, in confidence, to the independent senior appraiser. It may also be seen by the PCT education lead.

To conclude the appraisal discussion by assisting the appraisee to set down, as an action plan, the agreements which have been reached and provide ongoing support for reviewing and updating personal development plans.

To agree a date to undertake an appraisal review six months following each appraisal to discuss progress towards achievement of personal development plans and provide further assistance if required.

To identify any areas where separate peer review by colleagues with relevant expertise and knowledge is required and agree the necessary arrangements, taking account of any such feedback in the appraisal summary.

To undertake all approved appraisal training, attend regular appraisal support meetings and be prepared to be appraised as an appraiser. Professional support to be provided by appraisal support group. Appraisers will participate in the appraisal evaluation programme.

To recognise potentially serious performance issues where a colleague's health, conduct or performance poses a threat to patients. It would be exceptional for such serious concerns to be first identified at appraisal, but both appraisers and appraisees need to recognise that as registered medical practitioners, patients must be protected. (GMC *Good Medical Practice*, paragraphs 26 to 28).

To comply with the requirements of the Data Protection Act in respect to the storing and use of all appraisal documentation and to undertake to return all such documentation should your role as appraiser cease.

TO BE PROVIDED BY THE PCT
Contact details will be provided by the appraisal administrator in order for the appraiser and appraisee to liaise and agree appraisal dates.

Paperwork will be sent to the appraisee at least two months prior to appraisal.

The appraisal venue will be agreed between appraiser and appraisee. The PCT will endeavour to provide appropriate accommodation if required.

The PCT will hold a register of appraisal appointments, and will inform the appraiser and the appraisee when a review is due. Dates for reviews will be arranged between appraiser and appraisee.

Training for appraisers will be arranged by the PCT and associated expenses incurred by GPs reimbursed.

Consideration will be given to supporting reasonable actions required by GP appraisers to meet their objectives and fulfil their personal development.

NOTICE PERIOD
Either side should give three months notice of their intention to terminate this arrangement.

HEALTH AND SAFETY
The PCT has an obligation under the Health and Safety at Work Act, 1974, to provide safe and healthy working conditions. You are required to co-operate with management in discharging its responsibilities under the Act and to take reasonable care for the health and safety of yourself and others.

PERSONAL PROPERTY
The PCT advises its staff that responsibility is not accepted for articles lost or damaged on the PCT's premises, whether by fire, theft or otherwise; with the exception of money or valuables which have been handed to the PCT for safe custody and for which a receipt has been given.

CONFIDENTIALITY
Information concerning patients and staff is confidential and must not be disclosed to any unauthorised persons. In instances where it is found that a member of staff has disclosed any such information this could result in disciplinary action being taken against them. The Data Protection Act 1984 also renders an individual liable for prosecution in the event of unauthorised disclosure of electronically stored information. A breach of confidence could also result in a civil action for damages.

EQUAL OPPORTUNITIES
You are advised at all times to carry out your responsibilities with due regard to the PCT's equal opportunities policy.

CONFLICT OF INTEREST
In accordance with the PCT's conflict of interest policy you must declare to the PCT any financial interest or relation you may have which may affect the PCT's policy or decisions.

INDEMNITY
The appraiser will be indemnified, through the PCT's indemnity scheme, against any claims arising from their role as appraiser, so long as any such claims arise out of the proper execution of their duties and the appraiser has complied with the Central Cheshire PCT appraisal policy and procedures.

Signed . . . .
(for Central Cheshire Primary Care Trust)

Date . . . .

Acceptance
I accept the terms and conditions as set out in this letter of appointment.

Signed . . . .

Date . . . .

Specimen appraisal evaluation form for appraisee to complete

Example 1. Adapted from the National Clinical Governance Support Team model[1]

1 Very poor/ly	2 Poor/ly	3 Average/ly	4 Good/Well	5 Very good/Well

The trust's approach to appraisal   *1   2   3   4   5*

The trust's approach to appraisal is
The trust's support of me in addressing my developmental needs
How well were you able to complete the development plan in last
    year's appraisal?
The trust's response to general issues arising out of appraisal

My appraiser's skills   *1   2   3   4   5*

The appraiser's skill in conducting my appraisal
My preparation for appraisal was
The appraiser's preparation for the appraisal was
Your appraiser's ability to listen to you
The appraiser was supportive
The appraiser made me think about new areas for development
My overall rating of my appraiser in their role as an appraiser

The appraisal interview   *1   2   3   4   5*

Usefulness of the appraisal in your professional development
The appraiser reviewed progress against last year's development
   plan
How challenging was the appraisal in making me think about my
   practise
The development plan reflects my main priorities for development
My appraisal was worthwhile

The administration of appraisal   *1   2   3   4   5*

Forms and material to prepare for appraisal were available
I was given adequate notice of my appraisal
The process for allocation of my appraiser allowed me an element of
   choice
My confidence in the confidentiality of the appraisal
Time available to prepare for the appraisal interview

My overall rating of the administration supporting appraisal in the trust

> Comments of how the trust could improve its approach to appraisal
>
>
>
> Comments to help your appraiser improve their skills
>
>
>
>
> How could you or your appraiser have made the appraisal interview more successful?
>
>
>
>
> How could the administration of appraisal and support of appraisal be improved?

Example 2. Adapted from the Essex Model[2]

TO APPRAISER: Please hand this questionnaire to your appraisee at the end of the appraisal for completion, in confidence, subsequent to the actual appraisal.

TO APPRAISEE: We would be very grateful if you would please take the time to complete the following questionnaire. Please be assured that the questionnaire will be dealt with in the strictest of confidence and will be anonymous. The results of the questionnaire will be used to influence future appraiser training and selection and will not form any part of your appraisal.

Where appropriate, please write in block capitals. Please put an **x** in the appropriate box to indicate your answer/opinion.

Name of appraiser:

Appraisee's PCT:

ADMINISTRATIVE SUPPORT FOR YOUR APPRAISAL

	Strongly agree	Agree	Neutral	Disagree	Strongly Disagree
1 I found the process for arranging my appraisal clear and easy to follow	☐	☐	☐	☐	☐
2 The lists of appraisers for my PCT were accessible to me	☐	☐	☐	☐	☐
3 I found the EQUIP website a good resource for my appraisal	☐	☐	☐	☐	☐
4 I felt supported by EQUIP/sessional GP team through my appraisal	☐	☐	☐	☐	☐

PRE-APPRAISAL PREPARATION
(collecting the data and completing the forms)

5 How long did pre-appraisal preparation take you?	Hours: ☐	Mins: ☐
6 How long did pre-appraisal take others (e.g. practice manager)?	Hours: ☐	Mins: ☐
7 Did you use the NHS Appraisal Toolkit?	Yes: ☐	No: ☐
8 Did you use another computer-based system?	Yes: ☐	No: ☐

If you answered yes to question 8, please give details ☐

	Strongly agree	Agree	Neutral	Disagree	Strongly Disagree
9 Pre-appraisal preparation was useful to me	☐	☐	☐	☐	☐
10 Completing the forms caused me to reflect on my practice	☐	☐	☐	☐	☐
11 Much of the pre-appraisal preparation can be done by practice staff	☐	☐	☐	☐	☐
12 The pre-appraisal documents were useful during the appraisal discussion	☐	☐	☐	☐	☐

THE APPRAISAL INTERVIEW

13 How long did the appraisal interview take?   Hours: ☐   Mins: ☐

	Strongly agree	Agree	Neutral	Disagree	Strongly Disagree
14 The appraisal interview was well structured	☐	☐	☐	☐	☐
15 The appraiser was well prepared and had obviously read Forms 1–3	☐	☐	☐	☐	☐
16 I felt able to discuss issues that were important to me	☐	☐	☐	☐	☐
17 The appraisal discussion caused me to reflect on my practice	☐	☐	☐	☐	☐
18 The time spent on the appraisal discussion was appropriate	☐	☐	☐	☐	☐
19 I found the appraiser was a good listener	☐	☐	☐	☐	☐
20 I found the appraiser's comments helpful and appropriate	☐	☐	☐	☐	☐
21 I felt comfortable during the appraisal discussion	☐	☐	☐	☐	☐
22 I thought the appraisal discussion rigorous	☐	☐	☐	☐	☐

APPRAISAL FEEDBACK

23 How long did post-interview feedback and completion of Form 4 and PDP take?   Hours: ☐   Mins: ☐

24 How long after the interview did you receive the feedback?   Immediate ☐   Up to 1 week ☐   Up to 1 month ☐   Longer ☐

	Strongly agree	Agree	Neutral	Disagree	Strongly Disagree
25 The post appraisal feedback was clear and well structured	☐	☐	☐	☐	☐
26 The feedback was helpful	☐	☐	☐	☐	☐
27 The feedback was appropriate	☐	☐	☐	☐	☐
28 The time spent on feedback was adequate	☐	☐	☐	☐	☐
29 The feedback helped me to formulate a clear personal development plan	☐	☐	☐	☐	☐
30 The post-appraisal document (Form 4) was an appropriate summary	☐	☐	☐	☐	☐

31 Have you arranged to have a further mid-year review?   Yes: ☐   No: ☐

Don't consider necessary: ☐

32 Would you choose this appraiser again?   Yes: ☐   No: ☐

If you answered no to question 32, why not?

	1	2	3	4	5
33 Overall, how would you score this appraisal on a score of 1–5?	☐	☐	☐	☐	☐

 1 = that you found the appraisal unhelpful and it did not cause you to reflect on your practice
 5 = you found the appraisal extremely helpful and thought provoking

Any further comments you may have on the appraisal system and your experiences of it (please use an additional sheet of paper if necessary)

Thank you for taking the time to complete this questionnaire. Please return it in the prepaid envelope.

Appraisal evaluation form for appraiser to complete

These forms are not in universal use but do allow issues to be explored when the appraiser and appraisee have very different views of the appraisal process. Clearly the form needs to address similar areas to the appraisee form in order for this comparison to be made.

Example 1. Adapted from South and East Dorset PCT

1 Strongly agree	2 Agree	3 Neutral	4 Disagree	5 Strongly disagree

---

Organisation of appraisal   *1 2 3 4 5*

I was given adequate notice to allow preparation for the appraisal
I received contact details for the appraisee
I knew where to get copies of the appraisal documents and forms
I received forms in adequate time to allow me to prepare for the
    appraisal
I was happy with the venue arranged for the appraisal
I am happy about the confidentiality of the appraisal process

My role as an appraiser   *1 2 3 4 5*

I discussed the content of the appraisal with the GP beforehand
I had prepared well for the appraisal
I tried to put the GP at his or her ease
I was able to challenge the GP to the appropriate degree
I found this appraisal difficult to manage
Summary forms were agreed and are an accurate record of what we
    discussed
The development plan reflects the GP's main priorities for
    development

The appraisal   *1 2 3 4 5*

The GP appeared to find it useful
The appraisal helped me identify new skills I need as an appraiser
    (detailed below)
The appraisal helped me identify new skills I need in my clinical
    work

Comments on organisation of appraisal

The PCT's role

The appraisee

My role

Comments on the appraisal itself

The appraisal lasted . . . hours

Specimen example of health checklist and sign-off statement

GP health checklist

Note: This is not about your appraisal. This is about collecting the right information to make sure that it is all in place when it comes to your turn for revalidation.

All that is required is a simple statement that you have considered your health needs on an annual basis, and taken appropriate steps to ensure they do not impinge on patient care, i.e. are you registered with a GP outside your own practice? Have you had your hepatitis B status checked?

If you have got a health issue that you consider significant:

- have the issues raised by an illness or disability been discussed with your own doctor or the occupational health service?
- are the appropriate people aware of them (e.g. partners, in some cases patients)?
- what safeguards are in place to ensure that your health problem does not interfere with your ability to carry out the full range of duties?
- what safeguards are in place to ensure that in those areas where it is impossible for you to carry out the full range of duties the safety of your patients is protected?

Are you able to make an appropriate statement about your health?

> e.g. Having carefully read the criteria for an unacceptable GP in *Good Medical Practice for GPs* (September 2002), I am confident that my health is not an issue that affects patient care.

Signed:... Date:....................

Having carefully read the criteria for an unacceptable GP in *Good Medical Practice for GPs* I am confident that my health is not an issue that affects patient care (or, there are safeguards in place to ensure that my health does not affect patient care).

Signed:... Date:....................

References

1 National Clinical Governance Support Team. *Assuring the Quality of Medical Appraisal: report of the NHS Clinical Governance Support Team Expert Group*. Leicester: NCGST; 2005.
2 Essex Appraisal Steering Group. *GP Appraisal in Essex: the Essex scheme*. Chelmsford: Essex Appraisal Steering Group; 2002.

Index

Page numbers in *italic* refer to tables.

T - #0661 - 101024 - C0 - 246/174/11 - PB - 9781846190834 - Gloss Lamination